Laparoscopic Cholecystectomy

*Difficult Cases &
Creative Solutions*

Laparoscopic Cholecystectomy

Difficult Cases & Creative Solutions

Avram M. Cooperman, M.D., F.A.C.S.
Director of Surgery, St. Clare's Hospital;
Professor of Surgery, New York Medical College,
New York, New York

ILLUSTRATORS
Jeffrey Cooperman
David Cooperman
Lisa Feldman

with 214 illustrations, including 100 in color

QMP

QUALITY MEDICAL PUBLISHING, INC

ST. LOUIS, MISSOURI
1992

Printed in the United States of America.

PUBLISHER   Karen Berger

PROJECT MANAGER   Linda Kocher

PRODUCTION   Judy Bamert, Kay Ehsani, Susan Trail

BOOK DESIGN   Susan Trail

COVER DESIGN   Diane M. Beasley

Quality Medical Publishing, Inc.
2086 Craigshire Drive
St. Louis, Missouri 63146

LIBRARY OF CONGRESS CATALOGING IN PUBLICATION DATA

Cooperman, Avram M., 1939-
      Laparoscopic cholecystectomy : difficult cases & creative
  solutions / Avram M. Cooperman.
          p. cm.
      Includes bibliographical references and index.
      ISBN 0-942219-28-7 (hardcover) — ISBN
  0-683-14521-5 (internat'l)
      1. Cholecystectomy. 2. Laparoscopic surgery. I. Title.
      [DNLM: 1. Cholecystectomy—methods. 2. Peritoneoscopy. WI 750
  C778L]
  RD546.C68 1992
  617.5'56—dc20
  DNLM/DLC
  for Library of Congress   91-38831
                                                              CIP

QM/LS/WZ
5   4   3   2   1

In dedication to
things that matter in life

family, love, faith,
integrity, industry, the environment,
charity, and humaneness

may the commitment be renewed
with enthusiasm

Preface

More than half of the 500,000 cholecystectomies done annually in the United States will be performed laparoscopically in 1992. In the future it is forecast that 90% of patients scheduled for gallbladder operations will be treated laparoscopically.

Laparoscopic pelvic surgery has been with us for more than 30 years. Acceptance was slow, to say the least. Once video chips and projection of magnified images became available, the popularity of laparoscopic surgery increased. Next, orthopedic surgeons and very recently general surgeons adopted it. Since the first laparoscopic cholecystectomies were performed in France in 1987 and in the United States in 1988, the initial public support has become a ground swell of public demand. Such a response to a new abdominal procedure has been unprecedented in general surgery. Apparently patient intolerance of the lingering incisional discomfort after open cholecystectomy or even the less disabling mini-cholecystectomy was underestimated by the medical community.

The public's demand for laparoscopic cholecystectomy has produced an unusual series of events. Patient insistence for this operation has meant acquiescence to a new and unknown methodology and forsaking a favorite standard operation. Many surgeons were comfortable and familiar with open cholecystectomy and satisfied with the results achieved. They were skeptical about this new operative technique and reluctant to be forced into an unfamiliar operative field in which the gallbladder cannot be directly visualized or palpated. It was left to young, community-based and academic surgeons to take the lead in this rapidly growing field, as evidenced by glancing at the contents of the new journals and books on laparoscopy. Thus the largest experience to date has been accumulated by a few surgeons who were instrumental in developing techniques and instruments for this emerging specialty.

Laparoscopic abdominal surgery is not an issue; it is a reality, fueled by the consumer. Once surgeons were forced to accept this fact, the field became so diluted that it is now difficult to gain the necessary skills and experience to ensure performance standards. Hospital administrators, eager to show that quality assurance standards were established, set arbitrary guidelines for privileging. Credentialing often became a political issue, and criteria varied among institutions and from community to community. Many institutions tried to hastily compensate for delays in starting laparoscopy programs. In addition, the unprecedented acceptance of laparoscopic surgery has pressured many surgeons to offer this treatment option before developing sufficient expertise. As a consequence, many gallbladders that should be removed by open techniques are pursued for 4 or more hours laparoscopically. Although conversion to an open cholecystectomy is a fail-safe alternative, it is used far too often intraoperatively because of misdeeds and technical errors rather than as an anticipatory maneuver. An otherwise routine cholecystectomy is often made difficult.

Laparoscopic Cholecystectomy: Difficult Cases & Creative Solutions is the outgrowth of my initial experience with over 300 consecutive operations plus teaching and observing these techniques at many courses and hospitals. This book is written for all who are engaged in this exciting new method of gallbladder removal. I hope that it will help shorten the learning curve for the novice and simplify difficult clinical situations encountered by the more experienced. Ultimately, if this goal is successfully met, this book should raise the comfort level of all surgeons performing laparoscopic cholecystectomy so that this operation becomes as routine as the standard set by open cholecystectomy.

For the reader's convenience this book is divided into three parts. Part I: Common Denominators details treatment options, equipment and instrumentation, and initial operative steps. An attempt is made to provide a comprehensive and unbiased survey of the instruments and equipment currently on the market. A prototypical operative sequence is presented and liberally illustrated to demonstrate the basics before the reader tackles the more difficult clinical problems presented in Part II: Problems and Part III: Complications and Outcome. The last two sections emphasize flexibility of approach in solving complex problems such as gangrenous gallbladders, common duct stones, and pancreatitis. Avoidance and treatment of trocar and needle injuries, complications of insufflation, and numerous other intraoperative misadventures are also analyzed.

A problem-solving approach pervades the book. Basic concepts explored in the first segments of the operative chapters are followed by graphic step-by-step depictions of the techniques used and case presentations using video images to document and substantiate essential points. Tips and tricks for avoiding pitfalls are scattered throughout these pages. Invited commentaries by experienced laparoscopists are included to provide the reader with additional perspectives.

Although training courses amply demonstrate that gallbladders can be removed safely from pigs, they offer a false sense of security to the surgeon. The clinical setting introduces the intricacies of anatomy and the pressures of operating on a live patient, who may present with various complicating factors. This book attempts to bridge the gap between the training provided in these courses and the intraoperative surprises often facing the surgeon. As readily as laparoscopy is now applied to biliary surgery, so it is finding selective applications for colonic, pelvic, and gastric surgery. It is imperative that all surgeons who wish to do advanced laparoscopic procedures, such as bowel resection, removal of liver cysts, hernia repair, and hysterectomies, first master laparoscopic cholecystectomy. Laparoscopic cholecystectomy is but a preview of events to come. The future promises broader applications of this technique for a multiplicity of patient problems.

Avram M. Cooperman

Acknowledgments

Jeffrey and David Cooperman enhanced the value of this work by contributing their illustrative talents and editing skills. Their artistic work proves that certain genes skip generations and then reappear in fine fashion. Their constant questions helped me to clarify my thoughts about many of the problems discussed in the text. The visual images presented will serve to frame a concise picture to complement the textual descriptions. I also thank Karen Berger, Carolita Deter, Linda Kocher, Susan Trail, and the rest of the staff at Quality Medical Publishing, Inc.; Josephine Alinea, a devoted indefatigable assistant, who revised the manuscript countless times; my office staff: Nancy Brown, Nancy Kaplan, Michelle Teitz, Caroline Brown, and Carol Silverstein; and the Lincoln Hospital surgical residents who helped develop our laparoscopic surgery program: Valerie Katz, M.D., Joseph Licata, M.D., Jaime Dorotan, M.D., Motria Ukrainskyj, M.D., and Hilde Jerius, M.D. Robert Bailey, M.D., from the University of Maryland, Department of Surgery, found the time to help us start our clinical program, and Steve Lefkovits and Peter Wu of *USA Today* helped computerize the video images. Lisa Feldman helped greatly with artwork and photographs.

The operating room staff at St. Clare's Hospital in New York has been an extraordinary group, devoted to developing and extending the techniques of laparoscopic surgery. Julie Jimenez, our innovative coordinator, continually devises technical modifications to facilitate surgery. Al Jackson, Sharon James, Lupe Ortiz, Cathy Villaluz, Sally Acosta, and Virginia Collazo, the operating room director, have also been enormously helpful.

The administrative staff and board of St. Clare's Hospital, especially Richard Yezzo, President, and Nicholas D'Agostino, Chairman, continue to encourage additional applications of laparoscopic surgery.

My medical school, Howard University, is always in my thoughts, as are the surgeons at the Mayo Clinic who provided encouragement, demonstrated patience, and exhibited great teaching skills during my residency. The surgical department of the Cleveland Clinic, particularly the senior associates George Crile, Jr., M.D., and the late Stanley Hoerr, M.D., fostered innovative thinking in abdominal surgery. It was a privilege to be associated with them.

Contents

III · Complications and Outcome

Laparoscopic Cholecystectomy

Difficult Cases &
Creative Solutions

·I·

Common Denominators

·1·

Treatment Options

Eight percent to 10% of the U.S. population, or 25 million people, harbor gallstones.[1] Every year, one million new cases of cholelithiasis are discovered and approximately 500,000 cholecystectomies are performed. Two thirds of the operations are elective and one third are performed as emergency procedures.[2] Gallstones are present at all ages. Less than 1% occur in patients under 20 years of age. The incidence between ages 18 and 39 years is 29%, between 40 and 59 years it is 32%, and in people over 60 years, the incidence is 39%.[3]

An increased risk for developing cholelithiasis has been associated with increasing age (three times), female gender (three times), obesity (two times), family history (two times), rapid weight loss (four times), and diabetes (three times).[4] These factors do not influence treatment.

WHO TO TREAT?

Most gallstones float harmlessly in bile and remain in the gallbladder. They are expelled during gallbladder contraction into the common bile duct and the duodenum. Only 2% to 3% of patients with gallstones become symptomatic each year.[5] Cholelithiasis tends to be a chronic problem that becomes apparent over years and decades, not over weeks and months. At any one time, 60% to 70% of patients with gallstones are asymptomatic. Nonspecific gastrointestinal symptoms develop in 10% to 30% of patients, and 5% to 10% of patients develop classic biliary symptoms.[4]

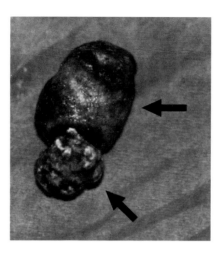

FIGURE 1-1 • This large stone consisted of two parts and completely obstructed the neck of the gallbladder (upper arrow) and upper cystic duct (lower arrow). This patient had nonspecific gastrointestinal symptoms and underwent surgery at the behest of her physician. Before surgery, I was uncertain that symptoms would be relieved. There was a large hydrops behind this large impacted stone that probably was present for years.

A careful history must be taken to determine if the symptoms are biliary related and if a cholecystectomy would be beneficial. It is not always a simple decision, particularly when abdominal symptoms are general and nonspecific. It is sometimes difficult to know when gallstones are asymptomatic and if nonspecific abdominal symptoms would be relieved after cholecystectomy (Fig. 1-1). Anticipated operative findings and laparoscopic findings frequently are at variance. There is usually a valid reason why gallbladder studies are ordered by gastroenterologists, even in asymptomatic or minimally symptomatic patients.

Once gallstones are detected, therapeutic options must be weighed. Not every patient requires treatment and certainly not everyone needs a laparoscopic procedure. Options and alternatives must be discussed with each patient.

Symptomatic Patients

The decision to provide therapy for symptomatic gallstones is not difficult. There is strong evidence that symptomatic cholelithiasis does not improve spontaneously but recurs frequently and at times with virulence. The complications of cholangitis, pancreatitis, and empyema may complicate the disease. For symptomatic patients, treatment is advised. Correlating symptoms with outcome facilitates the decision process.

Symptomatic gallstones present in several ways. When nonspecific biliary symptoms such as dyspepsia, bloating, and gaseousness persist, gastrointestinal studies should be performed. Often gallstones are detected. Since these symptoms are so prevalent and coexist with other intestinal maladies and stress disorders, many physicians have been reluctant to advise cholecystectomy in this situation for fear the symptoms will persist postoperatively. This fear may not necessarily be justified. In a recent series, nonspecific biliary symptoms were an indication for surgery in only 5% of candidates.[6] However, postoperative relief occurred in 75%. My experience confirms the favorable outcome in these circumstances, particularly when nonspecific biliary symptoms are of recent onset or represent a change from previous abdominal patterns.

The clearest presentation and indication for cholecystectomy is biliary colic with acute cholecystitis. In patients with classic postprandial or nocturnal upper abdominal pain, relief after cholecystectomy should be anticipated in nearly all cases. If symptoms persist after surgery, a common duct stone must be suspected.

Another presentation of cholelithiasis is typical biliary pain—but in atypical locations. This is due to referred pain or an enlarged or displaced gallbladder, which is the case particularly when the pain is in the right lower quadrant. Relief after cholecystectomy should be expected.

Some patients present with biliary-type pain or colic without documented gallstones. Gathering data about this patient group has been difficult. Examination and study by biliary scans during an episode of pain support the thesis that some patients have an obstructive disorder of the cystic duct, a motility disturbance of the cystic duct, or previously undetected gallstones. Objective confirmation of a biliary cause favors a good postoperative outcome with cholecystectomy.

When biliary-type symptoms exist without any objective parameters, caution must be exerted before proceeding with surgery since previous studies have not supported aggressive therapy in this situation. The laparoscope should make one no less vigilant about indications for biliary surgery. Many patients with biliary-type pain or colic have normal isotope flow through the bile duct but delayed or nonemptying flow from the gallbladder. Cholecystectomy benefits patients with biliary dyskinesia, particularly when objective data are present. This disorder is different from sphincter of Oddi dysfunction in which there is delayed excretion of isotope from the common duct. Patients with the latter disorder improve after sphincterotomy.

Asymptomatic and "At-Risk" Patients

An unresolved question remains about the performance of prophylactic cholecystectomy, both in asymptomatic patients and "at-risk" patients. The controversy has resurfaced with the new minimally invasive laparoscopic surgery. In patients with asymptomatic gallstones, the risk of acute cholecystitis developing is 2% to 3% per year.[5] In one study cholecystitis developed in 10% of asymptomatic patients with gallstones at 5 years' follow-up.[7] Although the chance of symptoms developing is minimal in any one calendar year, the risk is cumulative. Most patients correctly wait for symptoms to develop before seeking treatment. The risk of surgery is not increased by waiting for acute symptoms to develop. Thus for asymptomatic patients with gallstones, observation is wise. As a former colleague stated, "It is hard to make asymptomatic patients better."*

Gallstone patients considered to be "at risk" have included those who have diabetes or cirrhosis or who are undergoing surgery for other abdominal disorders.[8,9] The last patient group is the easiest to deal with. Cholecystectomy—laparoscopic or open—can be combined with any other intra-abdominal procedure. Gallbladders in these patients are rarely inflamed and are dissected easily and safely. This is a low-risk operation without sequelae, assuming the primary procedure has gone well. It may prevent cholecystitis from developing postoperatively.

In the diabetic patient with gallstones there has been concern that the septic complications associated with cholecystitis will be more severe and associ-

---

*Stanley O. Hoerr, M.D., a surgeon at the Cleveland Clinic, emphasized this point. It became known as Hoerr's Law.

ated with a higher morbidity and mortality. However, diabetes itself does not increase the operative risk of elective biliary surgery. In diabetic patients with cardiovascular or renal disease who undergo elective or emergency abdominal surgery, the risk posed by the surgery is no greater than that posed by renal or cardiac disease.[10,11] But until diabetic patients with asymptomatic gallstones can be guaranteed a zero percent morbidity and mortality after cholecystectomy, I do not think prophylactic cholecystectomy should be advised.

Another challenging patient group is cirrhotic patients with gallstones. Most often, the gallstones are bilirubinate and are secondary to low-grade hemolysis. When jaundice complicates the presentation, the issue of decompensated cirrhosis vs. common duct stones arises. The cause of the jaundice should be determined preoperatively with endoscopic retrograde cholangiopancreatography (ERCP). Cholecystectomy does pose an increased operative risk in patients with cirrhosis. Bleeding from the liver bed and unanticipated liver failure often develop. Since jaundice and abdominal pain in cirrhotic patients are just as likely to be caused by liver disease as by gallstones, prudent decision making and liberal use of ERCP is called for preoperatively. If doubt exists as to the origin of the pain or if the operative risk is significant, consideration of other procedures should be given (i.e., cholecystostomy with evacuation of gallstones, ligation of the cystic duct with cholecystojejunostomy, or endoscopic sphincterotomy alone).

ALTERNATIVES TO SURGERY

The patient with symptomatic cholelithiasis has several treatment options and must be made aware of them. These include observation, oral dissolution (with chenodeoxycholic acid or ursodeoxycholic acid), topical dissolution (with methyl *tert*-butyl ether), shock wave lithotripsy, and endoscopic or percutaneous approaches. Although all of these alternatives must be discussed in our litigious society, the ideal treatment for gallstones has always been to remove the gallbladder. It is the only procedure yet devised to avoid recurrent attacks of cholelithiasis. Cholecystectomy is safe and has a low morbidity.[12] The quest to develop nonoperative therapies has been based on a fear of surgery and the desire to avoid the pain and convalescence associated with open cholecystectomy. None of the alternative methods is definitive and all are associated with varying incidences of recurrent stones.

The results of a national cooperative trial on the treatment of gallstones with chenodcoxycholic acid at different dosages indicated complete dissolution of stones in only 8% to 14% of patients and partial dissolution in 27%.[13-15] Significant liver changes were noted in 3% and diarrhea developed in 8%. Ursodeoxycholic acid dissolution has been effective in 57% to 88% of patients.[16] Cholelithiasis recurs in at least 10% of patients who receive oral dissolution therapy.[16-18] The cost of and inconvenience involved with the medication, physician visits, sonograms, and other studies must be considered when the expense of oral dissolution therapy is calculated. Ideal candidates have a few floating small-sized cholesterol gallstones in a functioning gallbladder.

Contact dissolution with methyl *tert*-butyl ether provides rapid dissolution of cholesterol gallstones.[19-22] The catheter is placed transhepatically into the gallbladder and a precise system delivers and withdraws the solvent from the gallbladder. This system ensures that there is no overflow into the intestine. The complete dissolution rate can exceed 90%.[19-22] In one series, less than 10% of patients required cholecystectomy at a follow-up of 6 to 42 months.[20] The total treatment time averaged 12.5 hours and patients remained hospitalized for 2 to 3 days. Analgesics were required to control the pain from the catheter puncture site. The sole advantage of topical dissolution over laparoscopic surgery is that it requires only local anesthesia, which makes the procedure an option in very high-risk patients.

The introduction and success of laparoscopic cholecystectomy has caused research on and applications of electromagnetic shock wave lithotripsy to stall, and thus this form of therapy has not realized its full potential.[23-25] The start-up cost for equipment is expensive, the success rate for stone fragmentation variable (30% to 90%),[23-25] and the complications minor but not infrequent. The most common complication is biliary colic, which in some studies has occurred in up to one fourth of the patients. There are few lithotripsy units for the treatment of gallstones operating in the United States today.

Percutaneous extraction of gallstones by the passage of a guidewire and a catheter through the abdominal wall into the gallbladder to retrieve stones is also possible.[26-28] Fragmenting large stones by mechanical lithotripsy and then retrieving or basketing these stones is a modification of this technique. Multiple procedures and a hospitalization of several days are required.

An additional alternative has been to perform an ERCP-sphincterotomy and remove the common duct stones, leaving the gallbladder intact. This approach may be particularly effective when the cystic duct is not obstructed. Surprisingly few patients develop cholecystitis after the initial procedure and many continue to pass some gallstones of a large size.[29] This result indicates that addressing the immediate circumstance in biliary disease sometimes suffices, particularly in medically compromised patients.

Lest one believe that expensive biochemical manipulations or the use of technical aids are the only methods to treat gallstones, a study from China holds special interest.[30] Three hundred sixty-five patients with symptomatic gallstones documented by ultrasound and cholecystography were randomly treated by compression of auricular points. Three fourths of the patients were women. A hard seed, *Semen vaccariae,* was placed over the main auricular points for 20 minutes thrice daily after meals for 1 month. Each ear was used on alternate days and the seeds were changed every 3 days (to maintain hard pressure on the auricular points).

Stools were examined for stones. After treatment, gallstones were recovered in the stool of 299 treated patients (82%), in seven of 47 controls (15%), and in four of 45 cholagogue-treated patients (9%). Repeat ultrasonography after auricular compression revealed the stones to have disappeared completely in 5%, to be reduced in number by half in 56 patients (16%), and to be fewer in number in 72 (20%). In 127 patients (35%), the number of stones was unchanged, and in 69 (19%), the number increased. Stones were expelled more frequently from the common duct than from the gallbladder, and multiple small stones (<0.5 cm) were expelled from the gallbladder more frequently than single larger stones. The rate of expulsion was increased when the treatment was extended beyond 30 days. The real benefit of the acupressure treatment was limited to the 21% whose stones completely disappeared or were reduced in number by one half. Since this percentage is close to that of control patients who passed stones spontaneously (15%), was the benefit serendipitous?

The commentary and editor's note that followed the authors' summary cited five reports in the Chinese literature of studies using auricular pressure to treat gallstones, with success rates ranging from 37% to 97%.[31-36] The presumed mechanism is an increase in bile flow due to relaxation of the sphincter of Oddi and contraction of the gallbladder. Stones as large as 2 cm have been recovered from stools after acupressure treatment. A decrease in the size of the gallbladder has been documented by ultrasound after such treatment. In many areas of Asia acupressure is the first treatment for biliary ascariasis.

The editor concludes that "clearly, there is much to be learned. I, for one, would like to learn." This inquisitive open-minded approach applies to acupressure as much as to other biliary disease treatments.

CHOLECYSTECTOMY

Cholecystectomy has been performed for more than 100 years. A retrospective review of a large number of patients who underwent cholecystectomy at one institution over a 50-year period (including the preantibiotic era) indicated an overall operative mortality of 0.6%.[37] For acute cholecystitis, the mortality rate was 1.2%. When data for the last 7 years of the study were examined, the operative mortality was reduced to 0.2%, with the few deaths caused by cirrhosis and cardiovascular disease.

Today, procedure-related morbidity following open cholecystectomy is low: about 2%. These complications include bleeding, abscesses, bile leaks, or bile duct injuries. Bile duct injuries are the most serious and the incidence ranges from 1 in every 250 to 1000 cholecystectomies.[5,12,38] Open cholecystectomy is safe but is associated with incisional pain and a convalescent time that varies from weeks to months. Open cholecystectomy remains the standard against which laparoscopic cholecystectomy must be compared.

A modification of cholecystectomy, "Band-Aid" or mini-cholecystectomy, avoids division of muscle fibers and is associated with less pain and a shorter convalescence than standard cholecystectomy. A 3 to 5 cm incision lateral to the rectus muscle facilitates entry into the abdomen over the gallbladder. The common duct and sphincter may be explored through the incision (Fig. 1-2). The procedure usually requires a one-night stay in the hospital, but the

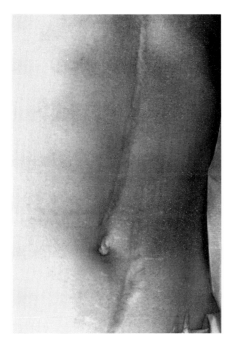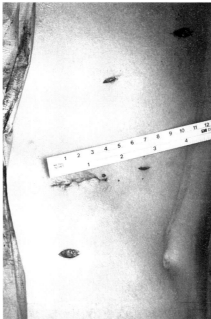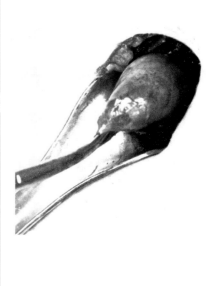

FIGURE 1-2 • This patient with multiple scars secondary to abdominal surgery was referred for laparoscopic cholecystectomy. Although pneumoperitoneum was successfully achieved through multiple port punctures, exposure of the gallbladder was difficult and an interface to dissect adhesions could not be found. Finally, the 10 mm lateral fundic port site was converted to a 3.5 cm nonmuscle-splitting incision ("Band-Aid" cholecystectomy) and the gallbladder was easily removed through it. The patient was dismissed 24 hours after surgery.

incisional pain can delay convalescence for 1 to 2 weeks.[39] It is now the fallback procedure when laparoscopic cholecystectomy is not possible.

LAPAROSCOPIC CHOLECYSTECTOMY

A small scar (cosmesis), less pain (comfort), a short period of bed rest (very brief to no hospitalization), and a quick convalescence (return to normal activity) are four reasons why laparoscopic cholecystectomy has been embraced by physicians, surgeons, and patients.

For the surgeon, the advantages of laparoscopic cholecystectomy are apparent early in a laparoscopic procedure when a chronically inflamed gallbladder is visualized at 18 times magnification without having to create a large

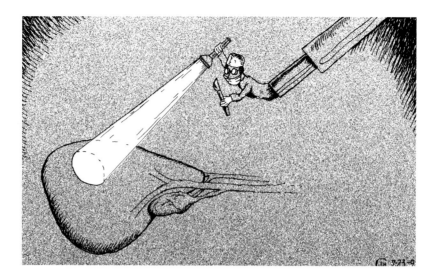

FIGURE 1-3 • The view of the biliary and hilar structures offered by laparoscopy lets the abdominal surgeon feel as if he is an integral part of the operative field.

abdominal incision (Fig. 1-3). For the patient, the benefits are obvious when the skin, fascia, and muscle are not transected. In traditional open cholecystectomy procedures the role of the surgical assistant was to provide traction and exposure from his "perch" above the liver. Rarely did he view or otherwise participate in the operation. In contrast, the view during laparoscopic surgery is shared by everyone in the operating room and little retraction is required.

The eye (in this case, the camera, attached to the laparoscope) is centered at the infundibulum of the gallbladder. Without retraction of the liver, duodenum, or colon, the gallbladder and cystic triangle can be exposed with minimal retraction. With a little dissection, the cystic duct, cystic artery, and lower common duct are clearly seen. The technical benefits of (1) magnification, (2) exposure of the cystic duct–common duct junction, (3) exposure of the lower and middle common duct, (4) clear view of the gallbladder, and (5) avoidance of a large abdominal incision place the surgeon in the center of the arena at the tip of the laparoscope, just inches from the hilum, with little effort.

With these advantages, certain concerns have been voiced. At first view, magnification can make one uneasy about the relative size of the cystic duct and cystic artery. There is a natural reluctance to clip a once friendly small structure that now appears formidable in size. By firing a 9 mm clip outside the body, looking at its true size, and then introducing the instrument to the operative site, the surgeon has established a reference point for size. In fact, the 9 mm clip makes the cystic artery look diminutive.

Although the laparoscopic view of the lower bile duct is excellent, the view of the hepatic duct and depth perception above the cystic duct are poor (Fig. 1-4, *A* and *B*). Many common duct injuries have happened at laparoscopy because structures cannot be adequately visualized. Direct identification of the cystic duct–common duct junction is thus mandatory by dissection and/or cholangiography.[40] Traction on the lower part of the gallbladder further distorts and tents the lower common duct, particularly from the perspective offered by the laparoscope since it is parallel, not perpendicular, to the lower common duct (Fig. 1-4, *C*). This view is opposite that achieved with open

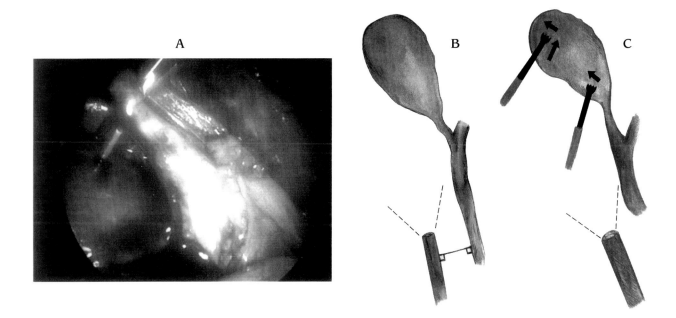

FIGURE 1-4 • **A,** This photograph depicts the difficulties with laparoscopic surgery. Although the view of the cystic duct is unequaled in terms of visualizing both its diameter and its junction with the common duct, the upper hepatic duct is not seen. With the camera at the umbilicus and upward traction on the gallbladder, the cystic duct–common duct junction is distorted. **B,** The misleading view is due to the fact that the "eye" (camera and laparoscope) parallels the common duct, rather than being perpendicular to it, which is the view achieved in open cholecystectomy. **C,** Traction on the gallbladder further distorts the view by tenting the lower common duct. This distortion and the lack of depth perception limit exposure of the hepatic duct.

cholecystectomy (Fig. 1-5) and can at first make orientation difficult and the perspective foreign.

The common duct, easily accessible at open surgery, appears alien through the laparoscope. Access is indirect (through the cystic duct), suturing is cumbersome, and tying knots laparoscopically is a new skill.

The awkwardness and inconveniences can be overcome with time, patience, and experience. This form of surgery is still in its infancy. With time, maturity and perspective will come.

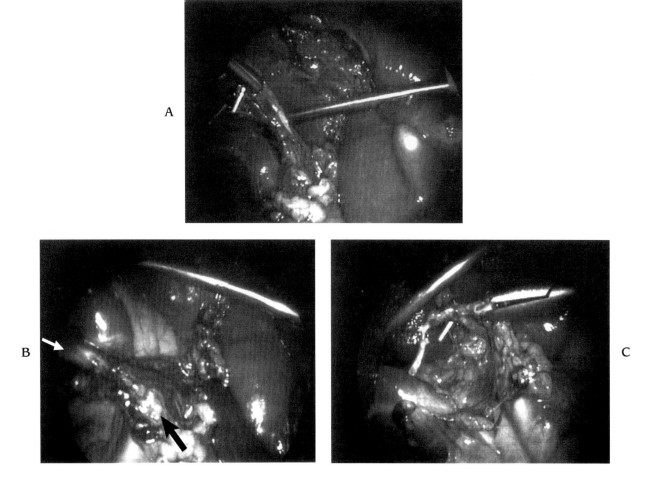

FIGURE 1-5 • **A,** The lack of depth perception and poor view of the hepatic duct, even when the liver is retracted upward by an instrument in the operating port, are frequent problems with laparoscopic cholecystectomy. **B,** When the camera is moved to the fundic port, the upper hepatic duct is seen and the distance between the cystic duct (white arrow), hepatic duct (black arrow), and liver is better appreciated. **C,** Rotating the cystic duct (in clamp) exposes the common duct in its length.

Other concerns include the dearth of available instrumentation for operating on "difficult" gallbladders, the significant delay in receiving ordered instrumentation, the high start-up expense of a laparoscopic surgery program, and the dependence on technical equipment and personnel in an operative situation in which nonfunction is synonymous with case cancellation or conversion to open cholecystectomy.

Selection of Candidates

Candidates for laparoscopic cholecystectomy must be candidates for both laparoscopy and cholecystectomy. There are no absolute criteria that exclude patients from either procedure. Fixed selection criteria for laparoscopic cholecystectomy tend to be too rigid and exclusive. Although multiple adhesions, ascites, pregnancy, and uncorrected coagulation defects may make laparoscopy difficult, in nearly all cases the laparoscope can be introduced and a decision about cholecystectomy can then be based on anatomic findings and the experience of the surgeon.[41]

The view that laparoscopy should not be done after previous abdominal surgery is unjustified. A recent report indicated that although the incidence of adhesions seen at laparoscopy was ten times greater in patients who had previous abdominal surgery than in nonoperated patients, the presence of adhesions did not alter planned pelvic laparoscopic surgery.[42]

Regarding cholecystectomy, there are few patients in whom a laparoscopic approach should not be considered. Patients with acute pancreatitis and suppurative cholangitis should have these disorders corrected before a laparoscopic procedure is attempted.

Although there is a natural reluctance medicolegally to perform laparoscopic surgery on a pregnant woman, particularly since most patients with cholelithiasis, pregnant women included, can be managed nonoperatively, pregnant patients have undergone successful intra-abdominal laparoscopic surgery, including cholecystectomy.[43,44] An operation or percutaneous drainage of the gallbladder is required infrequently for unrelenting acute obstructive cholecystitis. This situation occurs in less than 5% of cases of acute cholecystitis.

There has been much discussion about coagulopathies and laparoscopic surgery. This controversy is analogous to the issue of liver biopsy and coagulopathies several years ago. There were vocal advocates on both sides, but eventually good sense prevailed and now coagulopathies are corrected and closed or directed biopsies are done. Do small incisions bleed less than large incisions? Can bleeding be well controlled laparoscopically? These issues must be addressed on a case-by-case basis, particularly in the absence of any controlled trials. In most patients, the coagulation defect can be corrected preoperatively with blood products and the laparoscopic procedure can be performed with caution. If bleeding is significant or uncontrolled, the operation can be converted to an open procedure and completed.

REFERENCES

1. Strom BL, Tamragouri RN, Morse ML, et al. Oral contraceptives and other risk factors for gallbladder disease. Clin Pharm Ther 39:335-341, 1986.
2. Pickleman J, Gonzalez R. Improving results of cholecystectomy. Arch Surg 121:930-934, 1986.
3. Commission on Professional and Hospital Activities. American College of Surgeons, 1986.
4. Brugge WR, Atkinson HL, Lane BP, et al. Gallbladder dyskinesia in chronic acalculous cholecystitis. Dig Dis Sci 31:461-467, 1986.
5. Gracie W, Ransohoff DF. The natural history of silent gallstones: The innocent gallstone is not a myth. N Engl J Med 307:798-800, 1982.
6. Gilliland TM, Traverso W. Modern standards for comparison of cholecystectomy with alternative treatment for symptomatic cholelithiasis with emphasis on longterm relief of symptoms. Surg Gynecol Obstet 170:329-344, 1990.
7. McSherry CK, Ferstenberg H, Calhoun F, et al. The natural history of diagnosed gallstone disease in symptomatic and asymptomatic patients. Ann Surg 202:59-63, 1985.
8. String ST. Cholelithiasis and aortic reconstruction. J Vasc Surg 1:664-669, 1984.
9. Ouriel K, Ricotta JJ, Adams JT, et al. Management of cholelithiasis in patients with abdominal aortic aneurysm. Ann Surg 198:717-719, 1983.
10. Sandler RS, Maule WF, Baltus ME. Factors associated with postoperative complications in diabetes after biliary tract surgery. Gastroenterology 39:630-634, 1963.
11. Ransohoff DF, Miller GL, Forsythe SB, et al. Outcome of acute cholecystitis in patients with diabetes mellitus. Ann Intern Med 106:829-832, 1987.
12. McSherry CK. Cholecystectomy: The gold standard. Am J Surg 158:174-178, 1989.
13. Danzinger RG, Hofmann AF, Schoenfield LJ, et al. Dissolution of cholesterol gallstones by chenodeoxycholic acid. N Engl J Med 286:1-8, 1972.
14. O'Donnell LDJ, Heaton KW. Recurrence and re-recurrence of gallstones after medical dissolution: A long-term follow-up. Gut 29:655-658, 1988.

15. Marks JV, Lan SO. The Steering Committee and the National Cooperative Gallstone Study Group. Low dose chenodiol to prevent gallstone recurrence after dissolution therapy. Ann Intern Med 100:376-381, 1984.

16. Podda M, Zuin M, Battezzati PM. Efficacy and safety of a combination of chenodeoxycholic acid and ursodeoxycholic acid for gallstone dissolution: A comparison with ursodeoxycholic acid alone. Gastroenterology 96:222-229, 1989.

17. Bateson MC, Hill A, Bouchier IAD. Analysis of response to ursodeoxycholic acid for gallstone dissolution. Digestion 20:358-364, 1980.

18. Fromm H, Roat JW, Gonzales V, et al. Comparative efficacy and side effects of ursodeoxycholic and chenodeoxycholic acids in dissolving gallstones: A double-blind controlled study. Gastroenterology 85:1257-1264, 1983.

19. Allen MJ, Borody TJ, Bugliosi TF, et al. Cholelitholysis using methyl tertiary butyl ether. Gastroenterology 88:122-125, 1985.

20. Thistle JL, May GR, Bender CE, et al. Dissolution of cholesterol gallbladder stones by methyl *tert*-butyl ether administered by percutaneous transhepatic catheter. N Engl J Med 320:633-638, 1989.

21. vonSonnenberg E, Casola G, Zakko SF. Gallbladder and bile duct stones: Percutaneous therapy with primary MTBE dissolution and mechanical methods. Radiology 169:505-509, 1988.

22. Zakko SF, Hofmann AF, Schteingart C, et al. Percutaneous gallbladder stone dissolution using a microprocessor assisted solvent transfer (MAST) system. Gastroenterology 92:1794, 1987.

23. Saekmann M, Delius M, Sauerbrucj T, et al. Shock wave lithotripsy of gallbladder stones: The first 175 patients. N Engl J Med 318:393-397, 1988.

24. Neubrand M, Sauerbruch T, Stellard F, et al. In vitro gallstone dissolution after fragmentation with shock waves. Digestion 34:51-54, 1986.

25. Magnuson TH, Lillemoe KD, Pitt HA. How many Americans will be eligible for biliary lithotripsy? Arch Surg 124:1195-1200, 1989.

26. Gibney RG, Chow K, So CB. Gallstone recurrence after cholecystolithotomy. AJR 153:287-289, 1989.

27. Picus D, Marx MV, Hicks ME, et al. Percutaneous cholecystolithotomy: Preliminary experience and technical considerations. Radiology 173:487-491, 1989.

28. Hruby W, Stackl W, Urban M, et al. Percutaneous endoscopic cholecystolithotripsy: Work in progress. Radiology 173:477-479, 1989.

29. Siegel JH, Safrany L, Ben-Zvi JS, et al. Duodenoscopic sphincterotomy in patients with gallbladders in situ. Am J Gastroenterol 83:1255-1258, 1988.

30. Chen PN, Dong SR, Chen K, et al. Auricular pressure in the treatment of gallstones: A randomized clinical trial of traditional Chinese medicine. Hepatology 7:781-784, 1987.

31. Zhang ST, Sun JC, Rem PF, et al. Efficacy of pressure over ear points in the treatment of 150 cases of gallbladder stones. Chin Acupunct Moxibustion 5:244-246, 1985.

32. Teng K, Li YQ. Clinical analysis of drug embedded over ear points combined with body needling in treatment of 100 cases of cholecystitis and cholelithiasis. Chin J Integr Tradit West Med 6:111-113, 1986.

33. Zhang YL, Yuan H, Liu SL. Analysis of pressure over ear points in treatment of 120 cases of biliary stones. J Tradit Chin Med 26:195-196, 1985.

34. Zhang R, Ma SZ, Zhang DC. The influence of ear point pressure method in gallstones expulsion and contraction of the gallbladder. J Tradit Chin Med 27:184-186, 1986.

35. Cooperative Group of Acupuncture Therapy of Gallstones of Yien-Tai, San Dong Province. Preliminary study on mechanism of action of biliary calculi expulsion by electro-acupuncture of riyue and qimen. J Mod Med Herbs 8:352-353, 1977.

36. Cooperative Group of Acupuncture Therapy of Gallstones of Wendeng, San Dong Province. Therapeutic efficacy of electro-acupuncture of riyue, qimen points in treatment of 219 cases of cholelithiasis. J Mod Med Herbs 8:349-351, 1977.

37. McSherry CK, Glen F. The incidence and causes of death following surgery for nonmalignant biliary tract disease. Ann Surg 191:271-275, 1980.

38. Madsen CM, Sorenson HR, Truelsen I. The frequency of bile duct injuries illustrated by a Danish county survey. Acta Chir Scand 119:110-111, 1960.

39. Cooperman AM, Siegel JH, Hammerman H, et al. Ongoing "threats" to biliary surgery [editorial]. Arch Surg 124:1368, 1986.

40. Cooperman AM. Laparoscopic cholecystectomy for severe, acute, embedded, and gangrenous cholecystitis. J Laparoendosc Surg 1:37-40, 1990.

41. Bailey RW, Zucker KA. Laparoscopic cholangiography and management of choledocholithiasis. In Zucker KA, ed. Surgical Laparoscopy. St. Louis: Quality Medical Publishing, 1991, pp 201-225.

42. Szigetvari I, Feinman M, Barad D, Bartfai G, Kaali SQ. Association of previous abdominal surgery and significant adhesions in laparoscopic sterilization patients. J Reprod Med 34:464-466, 1989.

43. Soper NJ. Laparoscopic cholecystectomy. Curr Probl Surg 28(9):593, 1991.

44. Schreiber JH. Laparoscopic appendectomy in pregnancy. Surg Endosc 4:100-102, 1990.

·2·

Equipment and Instruments

The procedure of laparoscopic cholecystectomy is still evolving, and much of today's equipment is being refined, rethought, or redeveloped. The technology and development of laparoscopic equipment are advancing so rapidly that in the short interval between the submission and the publication of this text, video equipment, imaging systems, and monitors may be further modified (Fig. 2-1). Some developments will be subtle, others striking. Systems that automate and synchronize color, light, and video are being refined. The addition of computers to "capture" a laparoscopic view on a hard disk and simultaneously reproduce it as a printed image in seconds is exciting and will soon be incorporated with operating room video systems.

Most laparoscopic instruments have been devised for pelvic and gynecologic procedures and are not suited for abdominal surgery. The entry of several new companies into this market will make specific instrumentation for abdominal surgery more available and less expensive. Ideally, laparoscopic operating instruments should be similar to those for open procedures, extended 18 inches, and modified to fit through the port. Laparoscopic retractors will soon be available. Their development will do much to increase the safety and scope of biliary, intestinal, and gastric surgery.

Devising extracorporeal and intracorporeal sutures, ties, and clips that will simplify approximation of the bowel is a priority. Their use could also be applied to other intra-abdominal procedures.

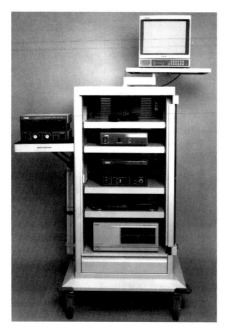 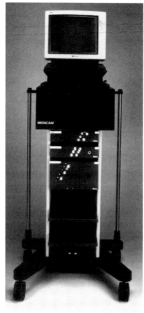 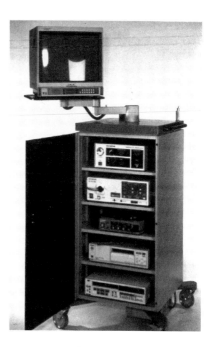

FIGURE 2-1 • Several laparoscopic systems are available. As design and technology continue to improve, the units become more versatile, compact, and less costly. Shown here are complete systems from Karl Storz Endoscopy, M.P. Video, Inc., and Olympus Medical.

INSUFFLATORS AND GASES

The basis of safety in all laparoscopic procedures is a cushion of gas delivered through an insufflator between the peritoneum and the abdominal viscera (Fig. 2-2). The pneumoperitoneum created allows ports and instruments to be introduced safely, permits the scope and camera to adequately visualize structures, and affords protection to the viscera beneath.

Many gases have been used to create pneumoperitoneum, including room air, oxygen, carbon dioxide, and nitrous oxide. The use of air and oxygen has been discarded because they pose a higher risk of embolism and are combustible with electrocautery and laser. Nitrous oxide is associated with the least degree of abdominal discomfort, but it does support combustion with cautery. Its absorption into the bloodstream is safe, but it is not as safe as carbon dioxide. Carbon dioxide is the gas most frequently used for insufflation during laparoscopy and has become the standard. Its great advantage is the very low risk of air embolism even when it is injected into the bloodstream (at quantities less than 1 L). It is noncombustible, harmless to the viscera, readily available, and inexpensive.

The delivery of gas through an insufflator has become more sophisticated. Present insufflators have digital gauges that indicate the pressure in the abdomen, the flow rate of gas into the abdomen, and the volume of gas insufflated. A current feature of insufflators is the autoregulation of gas flow to achieve a preset pressure with automatic resumption of flow if intra-abdominal pressure falls. As technology has improved, higher flow rates of gas have become possible. This is somewhat paradoxical since pneumoperitoneum is almost always achieved through a Veress needle, which, because of its small diameter and resistance, allows maximal flow rates of up to 2.7 L/min. For most procedures, once pneumoperitoneum is achieved, there is little need for high flow rates unless there is a major gas leak during the procedure.

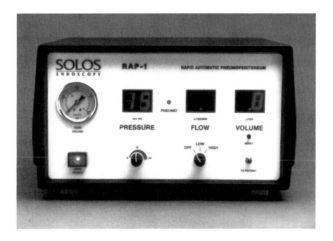

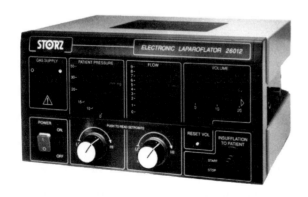

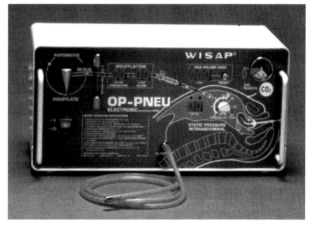

FIGURE 2-2 • Component pieces can be purchased to replace existing operating room equipment. Shown are insufflators from Solos Endoscopy, Karl Storz Endoscopy, and WISAP USA.

LAPAROSCOPES, LIGHT SOURCES, AND CABLES

Laparoscopes are essentially rigid telescopes. They have not been rede-signed in decades (Fig. 2-3). Most laparoscopes rely on the principle of light transmission along a quartz rod system. The system consists of glass rods with lenses attached at the ends. Laparoscopes are available in 3, 5, and 10 mm diameters. Objects can be viewed through a laparoscope end on (0 degrees) or at 30 or 50 degrees. Light is transferred through the scope from an external source without loss of intensity and without transfer of excess heat to the tip of the scope. Although the heat from the light source is intense at its origin, it is less so at the end of the scope because of the fewer number of optic fibers in the laparoscope. Heat transmission is further reduced by a shield that separates the light source from the fiberoptic cable and the fact that a significant amount of light is absorbed by the cable and not transmitted to the tip. Considering how frequently the light source is used, few mechani-cal breakdowns occur. A burned-out bulb is the most common failure experienced. The wattage of light sources increases with each new product. The need for a high-intensity light source is questionable. Like the high-flow insufflator, high-watt xenon light sources provide an intensity that is needed only when there is bleeding or a bile leak, both of which cloud the light in the abdomen. We frequently use 150- to 200-watt halogen systems; however, other available light sources also provide adequate illumination (Fig. 2-4).

Cables that connect the light source to the laparoscope are either fiberoptic or fluid. Fiberoptic cables are more commonly used and work well with the current xenon systems. Fiberoptic cables are theoretically less effective because they absorb a significant amount of light input and the blue and red parts of the spectrum are altered, making the true colors less vivid; however, this has not interfered with visualization during surgery. The fiberoptic light cable must be periodically checked to be certain that the fiberoptic bundles are intact. Fluid cables are less flexible than fiberoptic cables. Light absorp-tion is less and color transmission is better.

A new and welcomed feature is an automatic light control built into the camera or a manual control on the light cable attached to the laparoscope that makes it easier to modify the intensity of light. Operating room personnel are thus relieved from having to continuously adjust the light source.

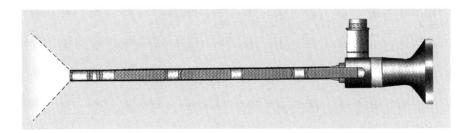

FIGURE 2-3 • An example of a rigid laparoscope: the Hopkins rod lens system.

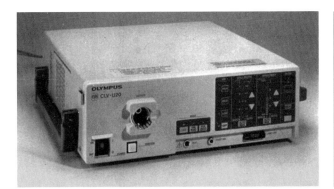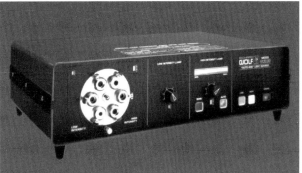

FIGURE 2-4 • Some available light sources.

Desired refinements for future laparoscope design include making the scope flexible, with channels for irrigation and instruments. A flexible laparoscope would allow "angling" of the tip to obtain multiple views of the bile duct. The addition of a rinse channel would allow cleaning of the lens without having to remove the scope.

CAMERAS

The "zen" of laparoscopic surgery is the production of a magnified reproducible image that can be immediately and simultaneously viewed by several observers. The continually evolving microchip technology has in a short time allowed camera development to advance from cameras with one microchip

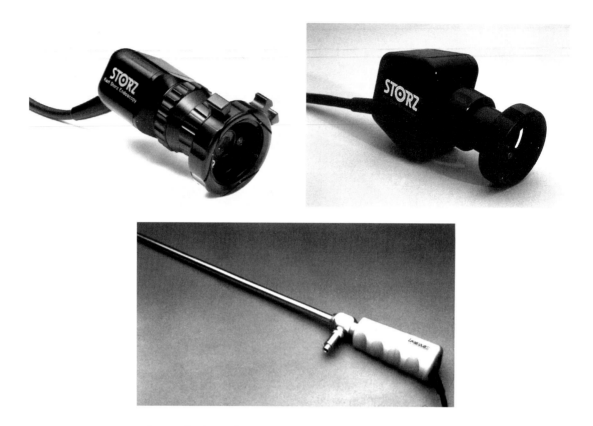

FIGURE 2-5 • The evolution of camera design from a single-microchip camera to a three-microchip camera to an enclosed unit.

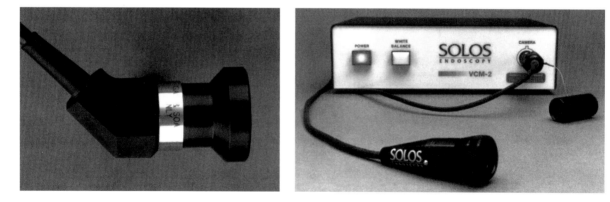

FIGURE 2-6 • Other available cameras.

(with a display of 450 lines of resolution) to those with three microchips (with a display of 750 lines of resolution) (Figs. 2-5 and 2-6). The camera attaches to the laparoscope and is joined to the video system by a connecting cable, which transmits the video image for viewing, recording, and printing. Once the images are balanced on a white background (white balancing), the new cameras automatically correct and adjust color and intensity. All cameras have manual adjustments for focusing and some have zoom features, which are rarely needed. Some new camera systems incorporate the camera and microchip(s) as a one-piece housed unit prefit to the laparoscope to facilitate cold sterilization. Although cameras may be soaked in glutaraldehyde (Cidex) or otherwise sterilized, their longevity is increased by avoidance of these sterilization modalities. The camera and upper cable are wrapped in a sterile plastic bag for every procedure and this practice does not alter the lens system.

Future modifications will include the addition of more microchips to increase the resolution and improve the sensitivity of the image, the ability to activate the recording and printing systems with controls on the camera, the adaptation of computers to seize and print frames, and the modification of the focal elements to allow automatic focus adjustments so that an even image is maintained throughout the procedure.

VIDEO MONITORS

Video monitors display the image optimally when their line resolution matches that of the camera. A camera that has 700 lines of resolution will not display the image well on a monitor with less than 700 lines of resolution. Conversely, a video monitor of 750 lines of resolution and a camera with 450 lines of resolution make for less than ideal image quality. Most monitors and cameras have 450 lines of resolution and are satisfactory for present needs. Monitors of greater resolution are worth the added cost only if they are used with a camera of similar resolution.

Monitors in the operating room differ little from those in private use but are three to four times the cost. Commercial monitors adapted to the operating room may be used, but all equipment should be grounded and approved for operating room use. The screen size should allow a clear, full image for easy visualization. The use of two 20-inch monitors permits optimal visualization.

Persons on each side of the operating table can maintain a direct line of sight. The length of the light cable limits the positioning of the monitor, thus the use of two monitors minimizes the distance between any one operating room team member and a monitor.

INSUFFLATION NEEDLES

To insufflate the abdominal cavity with gas requires the use of a needle or sheath of a port through which gas flows from the insufflator to the patient. A small-bore spring-loaded Veress needle is most commonly used for this purpose. First developed by Veress in 1938, the sharp needle has a spring that allows it to retract into the shaft after it punctures the abdominal cavity.

Insufflation needles can be disposable or nondisposable (Fig. 2-7). A regular sharp pointed needle could be used but it poses a risk of injury to underlying viscera. Disposable Veress needles have a clear plastic hub, which makes it easier to see the flow of saline solution into the peritoneal cavity when the correct placement of the needle is being checked. Since the unit is disposable, the tip of the needle is always sharp. Although some surgeons are concerned about the issue of needle sharpness with nondisposable insufflation needles, these needles can be reused effectively. Resharpening the point prolongs their usefulness. The use of nondisposable needles reduces the cost of instrumentation.

TROCARS AND PORTS

Once pneumoperitoneum is achieved, operating ports are placed into the abdomen. A port consists of an inner trocar and a surrounding sheath (Fig. 2-8, *A*). The trocar is used to puncture the abdominal wall and is then withdrawn, leaving the sheath to act as a conduit for the passage of instruments or gas. Seals or valves within the sheath allow the transfer of instruments without loss of pneumoperitoneum.

Several ports are commercially available. Like insufflation needles, they can be disposable or nondisposable. Besides the advantage of guaranteed sharpness, disposable trocars have a safety shield at the end. The shield

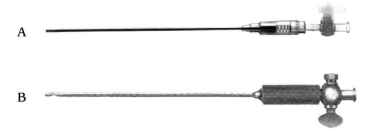

FIGURE 2-7 • Disposable **(A)** and nondisposable **(B)** Veress needles. A new modification is an optical catheter system that is attached to or threaded through a Veress needle, which provides a constant image during entry of the needle into the abdomen.

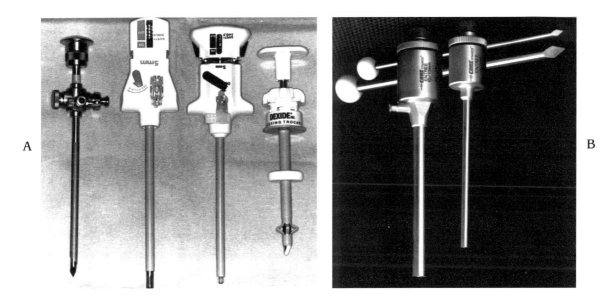

FIGURE 2-8 • The design and function of ports continue to be refined and altered. **A,** Five millimeter nondisposable and disposable ports. The evolution in design is shown from left to right. A nondisposable reusable port (Karl Storz Endoscopy), the United States Surgical port with a single valve, the Ethicon port with a seal and two valves, and the Dexide port are shown. The Dexide port can be secured between the fascia and abdominal wall by fastening the sliding disk above the skin and activating the umbrella device below the fascia. **B,** The newest entry to the port market from Core Dynamics consists of a nondisposable sheath with a disposable inner trocar. The manufacturer believes that this port design will reduce operating room expenses without jeopardizing safety.

retracts when the trocar pierces the fascia and then covers the trocar once the port enters the abdomen, thus protecting the underlying viscera. The retractable safety shield, however, does not substitute for careful surgical technique. As with all ports, the importance of a safe, nonforced entry technique into the peritoneal cavity cannot be overemphasized. Some disposable trocars are radiolucent, a feature that does not interfere with intraoperative cholangiography or fluoroscopy. Some ports are equipped with a gripping device that theoretically prevents the sheath from slipping out of the abdomen. I do not find these devices useful or necessary because if the ports are placed at a proper distance from the gallbladder, there is ample room to manipulate the instruments without altering the position of the port. In addition, the gripping device traumatizes the skin unless the incision is lengthened. With a new innovative trocar, port position is maintained by securing it both above skin level and below the fascia (Fig. 2-8, A). Another innovative port utilizes a nondisposable, easily sterilized sheath with a disposable inner trocar, which helps to reduce cost and to maximize safety (Fig. 2-8, B). My impression is that less force is required to puncture the fascia with this instrument.

As with nondisposable insufflation needles, nondisposable trocars can be reused repeatedly with safety. Resharpening the point prolongs their usefulness.

OPERATIVE INSTRUMENTS

If laparoscopic instruments were as plentiful as open instruments and designed similarly but modified to fit ports and extended 18 inches in length, there would be little difficulty operating on all gallbladders laparoscopically. Unfortunately, instrumentation is in such demand and short supply that it is sometimes difficult to obtain instruments. Companies have difficulties filling present order requests, let alone improving instrument design. The entry of other companies into this field will ease the burden of supply and facilitate surgery.

Operating instruments fall into one of three categories: graspers, scissors, and dissecting instruments (Fig. 2-9). With the exception of clip appliers and the large claw clamp, nearly every instrument fits through a 5 mm port.

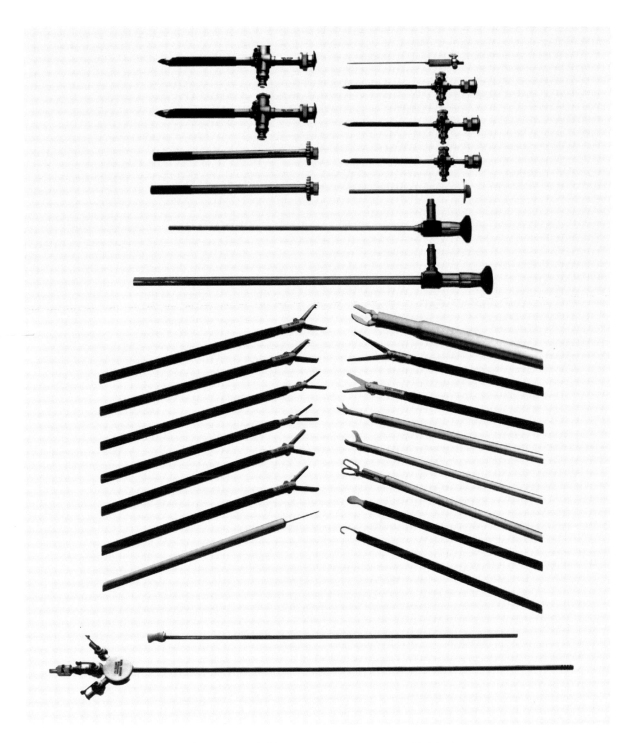

FIGURE 2-9 • Complete or partial instrument sets are available from several manufacturers. Shown are ports, laparoscopes, and nondisposable instruments from Karl Storz Endoscopy.

Grasping Instruments

Grasping instruments are used to secure and manipulate the gallbladder during surgery. Most have teeth too short to grasp the circumference of the gallbladder wall. For a thin-walled, nondistended gallbladder, nearly all graspers are effective (Fig. 2-10). For thick-walled and distended gallbladders, longer jawed, claw-type clamps are better suited (Fig. 2-10, *E*). Preferably, the clamp should secure the gallbladder without slippage and relieve the operator from having to maintain constant traction on the handles. Ratchet or spring-loaded clamps work well for this purpose. Clamps that will grasp the fundus and infundibulum without puncturing the lumen are ideal.

A common fault of most graspers is that their teeth are too short to effectively hold or manipulate most human gallbladders. They were designed for tubular structures in gynecologic surgery and are best suited for laboratory animal models of gallbladders. Some graspers have teeth that are too sharp and can puncture the gallbladder and cause bile to spill. Longer jawed, toothless clamps that distribute their force over a larger surface area are needed for laparoscopic cholecystectomy.

Scissors

Disposable and nondisposable scissors are now available. Nondisposable scissors are straight, micro, curved, or hook (Fig. 2-11). They can have single- or double-jaw action. Straight scissors are used for transecting the cystic duct and the cystic artery and occasionally for dissecting the gallbladder from the liver bed. Microscissors are used to cut fine structures such as openings in the cystic duct for a cholangiogram or to transect small ducts or arteries. Recently, curved Metzenbaum-type scissors were introduced for laparoscopic application. They are particularly useful for chronic thin-walled gallbladders but are less effective for thick-walled embedded gallbladders. The use of these scissors is ideal in institutions where laparoscopic experience varies among surgeons and there is the possibility that, in the hands of less experienced surgeons, the blades of nondisposable instruments may be damaged by improper use. Hook scissors allow a structure to be held in one depressed jaw of the scissors while the upper part secures and cuts it. The snout is blunt and less apt to injure contiguous structures.

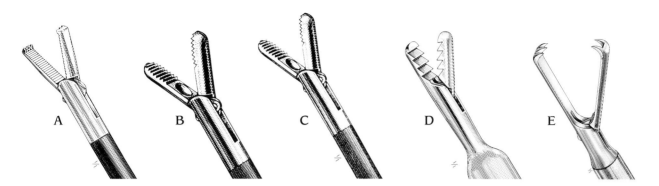

FIGURE 2-10 • Various grasping instruments.

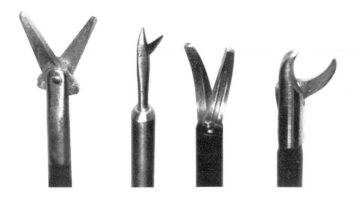

FIGURE 2-11 • Straight, micro, curved, and hook scissors. The curved scissors, a new product, are a disposable instrument.

Care must be taken with all nondisposable scissors to keep the jaws away from metal clips; contact will dull the blades and shorten the instrument's lifespan. If this precaution is followed, nondisposable scissors may be utilized without resharpening for hundreds of cases.

Manual and Automatic Clip Appliers

Single-clip and multiloaded clip appliers, whose clip diameter ranges from 9 to 11 mm (Fig. 2-12), contribute much to the success of laparoscopic surgery. They are used to secure vessels and ducts. Like manual ties, clips provide

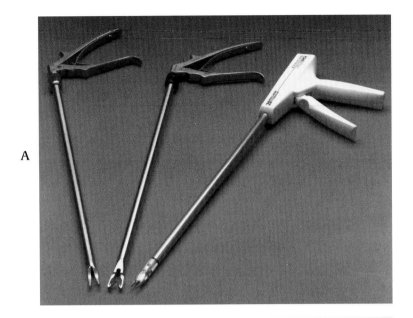

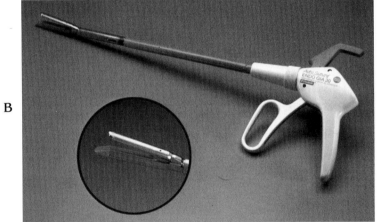

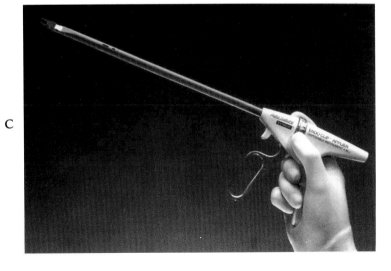

FIGURE 2-12 • **A,** Single-clip and multiloaded clip appliers. **B,** Soon-to-be introduced laparoscopic stapler that can secure and divide tissue automatically. **C,** United States Surgical clip appliers, the first multiloaded clip appliers.

secure apposition when applied correctly. The obvious advantage of the multiloaded instrument over the manual single-clip applier is that the multiloaded device does not have to be withdrawn through the port for reloading after each use. Since it is loaded in the abdomen, clip dislodgment is avoided.

Dissectors

Two instruments that facilitate laparoscopic surgery are the spatulated dissector and the hook dissector, the tip of which is curved or sharply angulated (Fig. 2-13). These instruments, the shafts of which permit cautery conduction, are used to dissect the cystic duct and the cystic artery and to free the gallbladder from the liver bed. In some dissectors the current is transmitted to the bottom of the shaft, thus "grounding" and cautery burn of the liver bed are common (but fortunately inconsequential). The spatula is a good blunt dissector and coagulator but a less effective suction/irrigation instrument because char accumulates on the tip and occludes the irrigating channel. It can be used to free the gallbladder from its bed, to cauterize adhesions, and to mobilize the cystic duct and cystic artery prior to ligation and division. In addition, when passed up and down behind the cystic duct, it can help to accurately locate the cystic duct–common duct junction. Most cautery tips are not insulated; the tip has a preset angle and grounds out in the liver bed. The commercial units are being modified to correct this. The handheld unit has also been modified to securely fit the sheath.

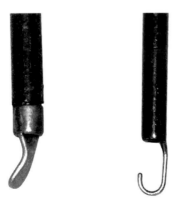

FIGURE 2-13 • Spatulated and hook dissectors with cautery insulation.

IRRIGATION SYSTEMS

To maintain a clear field and flush out blood or bile, several irrigating devices are available (Fig. 2-14). They range from 5 mm gravity-driven infusion systems to gas-driven high-pressure systems that deliver higher flow through 10 mm instruments. The uncomplicated inexpensive systems work well for most cholecystectomies. Efficacy is increased by adding a 28 Fr chest tube to the 5 mm suction irrigator and a pressure pump (blood bag) to surround the plastic liter container. Occasionally higher flow is needed to clear clots. Irrigation for this purpose is best provided by a high-pressure or gas-driven system.

A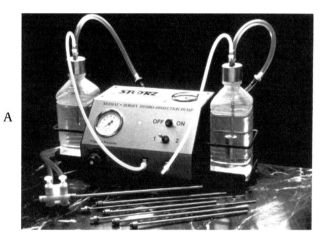

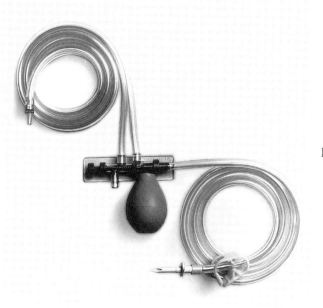 B

C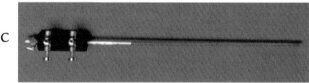

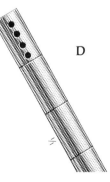 D

FIGURE 2-14 • **A** and **B,** Irrigation devices are gas driven or gravity flow. Trumpet valve controls **(C)** and irrigating tips **(D)** regulate inflow and outflow.

LASER OR ELECTROSURGERY

Both laser and electrosurgery have been used during laparoscopic gallbladder surgery (Fig. 2-15). Both use thermal energy to desiccate cells until the cells coagulate or explode (cutting current). A detailed discussion of laser and electrosurgery has been lucidly presented by Soper. Because monopolar cautery has been an operating room standard for more than 60 years, surgeons are more familiar with its use and risks than those associated with the laser. Electrosurgery is used in most laparoscopic cholecystectomies because it is significantly less expensive, is simpler to use, requires no training or credentialing, has a satisfactory safety record, and has a proven track performance.

Electrosurgery units are electrical generators that emit an alternating electrical current. The current may be adjusted by interrupting the flow (coagulation) or by maintaining a continuous flow (cutting current). When the modalities are combined, a blended current results.

The current produced reaches the tissue through the tip of the probe (active electrode) and is received at a remote site on the ground plate (return electrode). The current (electrons) courses through the body to the return electrode and, depending on resistance and voltage, conducts through other body tissues. It is essential that the patient be grounded on a secure-fitting plate and that low voltage is used.

Most electrosurgical cautery units are monopolar (the current returns to the electrode by flowing through the patient's skin). Thus there is a risk of burn injury to tissue and bowel. This risk of injury is avoided with the bipolar system since the paired connected probe tips serve to deliver the current through one tip and to return the current through the other. Bipolar cautery is available for laparoscopic surgery and works only as a coagulator, not as a dissecting instrument.

Although lasers were developed 40 years ago, they have become a more common fixture in the operating room only in the last decade. Lasers are very effective but are more expensive, require additional training, are slower, and are cumbersome to use. Safety measures, particularly eyewear, must be employed. Their advantages are their precision and predictability. Their use may become more popular as welding anastomoses and joining tissue become feasible.

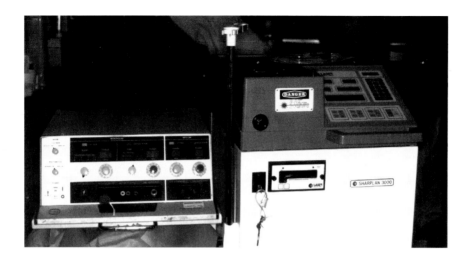

FIGURE 2-15 • An electrosurgical cautery unit (left) and laser (right).

Laser energy is created when electrons change their state of energy and produce photons. Photons then escape from a resonating chamber in a controlled fashion. Laser light differs from ordinary light in that the photons are of the same wavelength (monochromatic), are parallel (collimated), and are in synchrony. These combined qualities make laser light a more powerful energy source than standard light. The created laser beam may be scattered, reflected, absorbed, or transmitted through tissue.

For laparoscopic cholecystectomy, a neodymium:yttrium-aluminum-garnet (Nd:YAG) laser is often used. Infrared radiation transmitted through a quartz fiber and directed at tissue causes photocoagulation to a small zone (up to 6 mm). The addition of a contact tip to the quartz fiber (i.e., sapphire tip) focuses the laser energy on the tip, allowing a penetration depth of 1 to 2 mm.

Three other lasers are commercially available: the argon laser, the carbon dioxide laser, and the potassium titanyl phosphate (KTP) laser. They operate at half the wavelength of the Nd:YAG laser and produce similar tissue effects. The depth of coagulation is less than 1 mm when the fiber is held close to the tissue, and as the beam is withdrawn, the beam weakens. The beam of the carbon dioxide laser is collimated. This laser cuts tissue with very little coagulation, producing minimal tissue necrosis.

FUTURE HORIZONS

Despite the lag in research and design of laparoscopic instruments and devices, modifications of current devices and inventive new designs are being introduced to the marketplace (Fig. 2-16). Currently, unsophisticated instrumentation and difficulties in tying and suturing intracorporeally limit additional applications of laparoscopic surgery. As advances are made in the design of intracorporeal staplers, retractors, and instruments, laparoscopic surgery applications can be expanded to permit a wider range of intra-abdominal procedures.

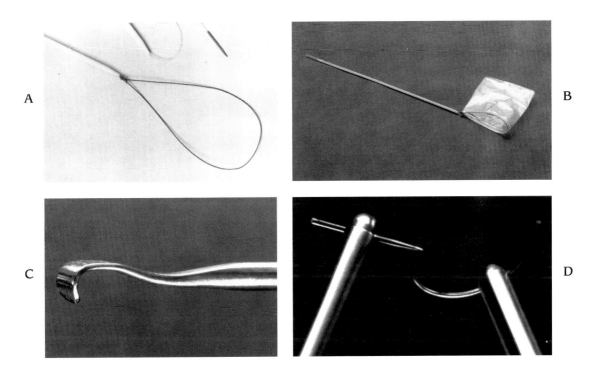

FIGURE 2-16 • Newer devices for laparoscopic surgery include pretied sutures **(A)**, bags to retrieve stones **(B)**, retractors **(C)**, and needle holders **(D)**.

Continued.

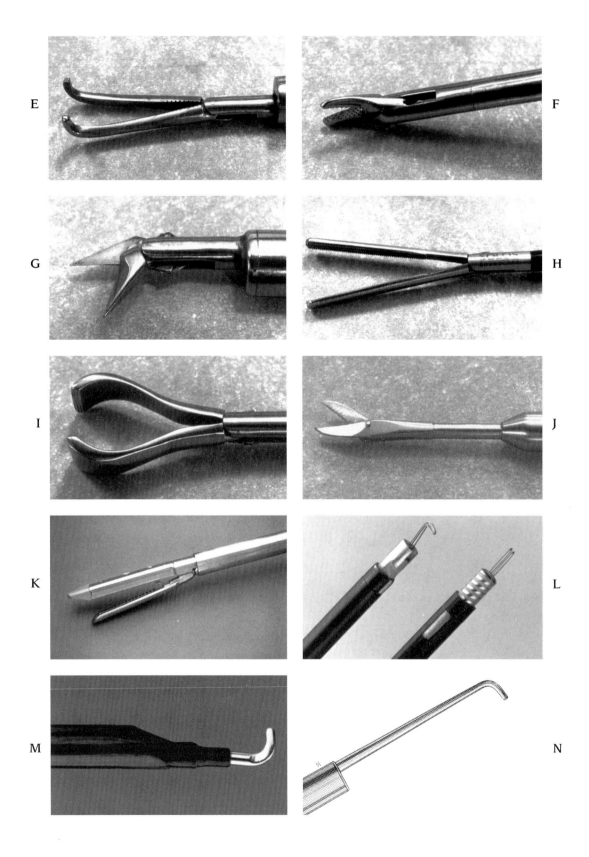

E

F

G

H

I

J

K

L

M

N

O

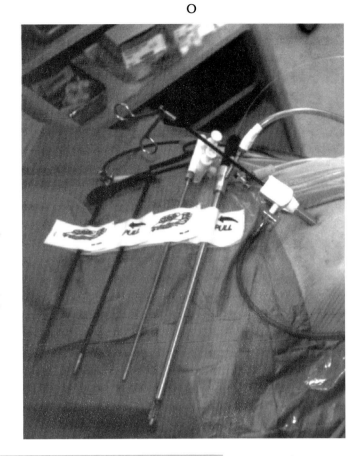

FIGURE 2-16, cont'd • **E-J,** Angled scissors, clamps, and needle holders are shown. Intra-abdominal laparoscopic surgery is also facilitated by stapling devices **(K),** bipolar cautery **(L),** and other refined dissecting instruments **(M** and **N).** Additional assistance can be obtained from Velcro devices used to secure lines and cords **(O). P,** New disposable electrosurgery hooks and spatulas with handheld cautery attachments have recently been introduced. Irrigation and suction channels are available (Aspen Laparoscopic Instruments). **Q,** New features include the adaptation of traditional surgical instruments, such as the Allis and Babcock clamps, for laparoscopic applications. These instruments from Weck include exchangeable or replaceable scissor heads.

P

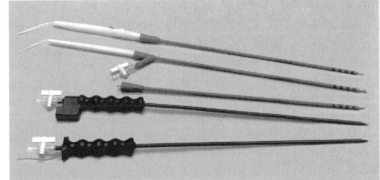

Q

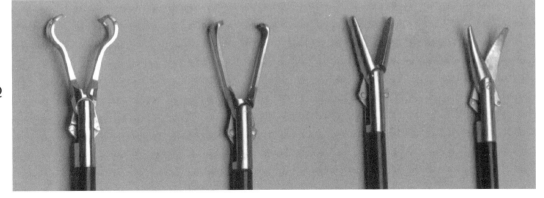

BIBLIOGRAPHY

American National Standard for the Safe Use of Laser in Health Care Facilities Z136.3 (1988). New York: American National Standard Institute, 1988.

Borten M. Laparoscopic Complications, Prevention and Management. Toronto: BC Decker, 1986.

Hasson HM. Modified instrument and method for laparoscopy. Am J Obstet Gynecol 110:886-887, 1971.

Hopkins HH. Optical principles of the endoscope. Endoscopy 1:3-27, 1976.

Hulka JF. Textbook of Laparoscopy. Orlando: Grune & Stratton, 1985.

Hunter JG. Laser or electrocautery for laparoscopic cholecystectomy? Am J Surg 161:345-349, 1991.

Riedel HH, Willenbrock-Lehnmann E, Mecke H, et al. The frequency of distribution of various pelviscopic (laparoscopic) operations, including complication rates— Statistics of the Federal Republic of Germany in the years 1983-1985. Zentralbl Gynakol 111:78-91, 1989.

Semm K. Operative Manual for Endoscopic Abdominal Surgery. Chicago: Year Book, 1987.

Soper NJ. Laparoscopic cholecystectomy. Curr Probl Surg 28(9):628-632, 1991.

Talamini MA, Gadacz TR. Laparoscopic equipment and instrumentation. In Zucker KA, ed. Surgical Laparoscopy. St. Louis: Quality Medical Publishing, 1991, pp 23-55.

Veress J. Neues instrument zur ausfuhrung von brust oder bauchpunktionen. Dtsch Med Wochenschr 41:1480-1481, 1938.

·3·

Initial Operative Steps

Once one has accessed the necessary equipment and instruments, familiarized oneself with their features, and obtained the assistance of a more experienced surgeon in laparoscopic cholecystectomy, one is ready to begin clinical operations.

SURGEON ELIGIBILITY

Much has been made about credentialing. At many hospitals it has benefited a select few. This practice is incorrect. What requirements should be fulfilled before soloing? Is animal experience necessary? Is previous laparoscopic experience a requirement? There are no absolute answers. The time-tested method of learning a new operation has been to observe it, assist during its performance, and then to be assisted by a more experienced surgeon. In laparoscopic surgery this learning sequence would require that a surgeon work with a laparoscopist (often a gynecologist), develop expertise by doing laparoscopy as a prelude to open laparotomy, and then assist and be assisted during laparoscopic cholecystectomy with a more experienced surgeon. This learning approach is ideal for resident training, and no doubt today's residents will be more comfortable with laparoscopic cholecystectomy than with open cholecystectomy. At our hospital a postgraduate fourth-year resident gathers sufficient experience during the surgical rotation to become adept at and be comfortable with performing the operation.

Gaining confidence and experience has been more difficult for practicing surgeons. They have limited time available for training. Consequently, a number of 1-, 2-, or 3-day courses sponsored by manufacturers of laparoscopic equipment have sprung up in the United States. These courses provide theoretical and hands-on experience. Familiarity with equipment and adaptation of hand-eye coordination while operating from a video monitor are the two immediate benefits of participating in these courses. However, the courses should not provide a false sense of confidence in laparoscopic ability and do not substitute for proctored experience.

Since standards for credentialing of other operations do not exist, privileging has been inconsistent. This has been a somewhat thorny issue. The guidelines by SAGES, the American College of Surgeons, and the Society for Surgery of the Alimentary Tract suggest that general surgeons (1) be trained in performing open cholecystectomy and be capable of managing the associated complications, (2) obtain laparoscopic expertise through clinical experience or instruction, (3) successfully complete a supervised experience in laparoscopic cholecystectomy including animal experience, and (4) notify patients of their experience with the procedure.[1]

At our small hospital, I assist any surgeon who wishes to do the clinical procedure. When we are mutually confident in the surgeon's ability, he then solos. This approach seems to be more sensible than arbitrarily selecting a fixed number of cases that must be done jointly. It has worked well and fosters a sense of cooperative endeavor among surgeons and the laparoscopic surgery team.

PERSONNEL

Once a large sum of money is expended on instruments and equipment, it behooves hospitals to develop a team of trained personnel and nurses to maintain it. A technician familiar with electrosurgery and video equipment should be on staff. He is then responsible for upgrading and maintaining the equipment to avoid costly repair, replacement, and delay. An intraoperative breakdown of equipment is synonymous with conversion to open cholecystectomy.

An experienced scrub team inspires confidence in the surgeon first learning laparoscopic cholecystectomy and allays anxiety during difficult intraoperative moments. In our hospital we initially assigned one nurse and one assistant to prepare and assist on all cases. When they were confident and familiar with the intraoperative sequence, they trained other individuals. In this way the hospital and personnel gained essential expertise.

PREOPERATIVE PREPARATION

After the presence of gallstones is documented and it has been determined that an operation is necessary, all cholecystectomy patients must undergo the requisite preoperative tests mandated by state law and hospital protocol. These tests include basic blood and chemical tests, liver function tests, and a coagulation profile. When the results of these tests are satisfactory and the physical examination is done, the patient is considered eligible to receive anesthesia. The patient is permitted nothing by mouth for 12 hours before surgery by tradition, but 6 hours or less is safe if only clear liquids are consumed. The patient reports to the hospital 1 to 2 hours before the scheduled operation. Patients are treated on an ambulatory basis or are admitted the morning of surgery. Insurance companies that only months ago were reluctant to reimburse for laparoscopic cholecystectomy are now vocal advocates of same-day admissions and ambulatory procedures. The length of hospitalization after surgery must be determined on an individualized basis. Whereas many patients can be dismissed a few hours after surgery, patients with pain or with complex medical histories are best kept overnight, insurance company requests notwithstanding. The patient is asked to sign an informed consent form for cholecystectomy that may be done either laparoscopically or open. The goals and risks of the procedure are again thoroughly reviewed with the patient.

ANESTHESIA

Laparoscopic cholecystectomy may be done with the patient under regional, general, or local anesthesia. The goals for induction of anesthesia are maximal patient comfort, a short postanesthesia recovery period, and few postoperative problems.

Since the abdomen is distended with carbon dioxide, an absorbable gas, pulmonary changes from both diaphragmatic displacement and blood gas exchange occur. These changes happen with every laparoscopic procedure and include increased levels of Pco_2 and alveolar carbon dioxide, and a decrease in pH, functional residual capacity, and pulmonary compliance. These pulmonary changes vary with the extent of diaphragmatic excursion, the patient's preoperative state, and the type of ventilation (controlled or spontaneous). All patients must be continuously monitored during surgery to correct any blood gas changes.

General Anesthesia

Most laparoscopic cholecystectomies are done with the patient under general anesthesia. The surgeon is most comfortable with this form of anesthesia, cardiac and respiratory status is best controlled, and ventilatory and cardiac problems are best prevented. It provides maximal patient comfort when carbon dioxide is used as the insufflating agent.

Regional Anesthesia

Thoracic epidural anesthesia is rarely used in laparoscopic cholecystectomy. The advantages of being awake are most appealing to the patient before surgery, but they are balanced by the need for intravenous sedation medication, which is associated with a risk of respiratory depression, to allay patient anxiety. Respiration and blood gases must be monitored carefully when the patient receives epidural anesthesia, particularly if the procedure is lengthy or complicated. For these reasons, it is used infrequently.

Spinal, Intercostal Nerve Block, and Local Anesthesia

These forms of anesthesia are almost never employed in laparoscopic cholecystectomy because they offer poor pain control and they make controlling respiratory changes difficult. When local anesthesia is used, less pneumoperitoneum must be insufflated to avoid patient discomfort. I suspect these anesthetic agents will become popular in the future when used in conjunction with gases other than carbon dioxide for insufflation and when the operation has evolved to the point where it will be done more quickly and routinely.

OPERATING ROOM SETUP

The standard operating room setup includes two video monitors, one on each side of the table, positioned towards the head of the table. They provide suitable viewing for all personnel in the operating room. The surgeon may stand on either side of the patient, but custom dictates a position on the patient's left. An alternative would be to place the patient in the lithotomy position and to have the surgeon operate from the foot of the table. Simplicity, comfort, and habit dictate which position is appropriate for each case. The camera operator stands next to the surgeon toward the foot of the table. To the patient's right side is the assistant, opposite the surgeon. The surgical nurse stands next to the assistant toward the foot of the table. The anesthesiologist and the monitoring equipment are at the head of the table. The laparoscopic and open cholecystectomy instrument trays are positioned at the foot of the table. This layout is fairly standard and conforms well to the space of most operating rooms.

OPERATIVE PREPARATION

Before the patient is placed under anesthesia, the camera, light source, scope, and insufflator should be checked to be certain that they are operational. The tank of carbon dioxide is also checked to ensure that an adequate amount is available for the duration of the operation. These precautions will reduce the chance of intraoperative malfunction and unpleasant surprises.

An intravenous infusion is started before surgery. A single dose of antibiotics effective against biliary organisms is given and the patient is positioned supine on the table with a footboard in place (Fig. 3-1). The footboard prevents unanticipated changes in patient position when the head of the table is elevated during the procedure.

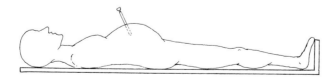

FIGURE 3-1 • Patient is positioned supine with footboard in place.

The abdomen is prepared with an iodophor solution that is applied and left for several minutes while the surgical team scrubs. The routine use of a nasogastric tube and Foley catheter is recommended when a surgical training program is first initiated; however, the stomach is rarely encountered during laparoscopic cholecystectomy and the bladder, when empty, is a safe distance from the umbilical location of the camera port. Therefore the practice of inserting a Foley catheter and a nasogastric tube may be done selectively. Patients are asked to void before surgery, which precludes the need for a Foley catheter, and if the stomach becomes distended intraoperatively (which is rare), a nasogastric tube can be passed.

ESTABLISHING PORTS

A transverse 1 cm incision is made directly through the umbilicus, and the subcutaneous tissue is bluntly dissected to the fascia with the knife handle or finger (Fig. 3-2). At the umbilicus the fascia and skin are in close proximity, which facilitates access to the peritoneum. The skin opening should easily accommodate the diameter of the port. The creation of an adequate-sized skin opening will limit the force necessary to penetrate the fascia. Some surgeons lift only the skin up before placing the Veress needle, but it should be the fascia that is lifted; this can be done with skin hooks (Fig. 3-3). This maneuver makes placement of the insufflation needle safer, particularly in thin patients in whom the abdominal wall is close to the retroperitoneal vascular structures. During this part of the procedure the patient is kept supine rather than in the Trendelenburg position because the small bowel is not displaced spontaneously by change in patient position. The Veress needle is placed obliquely through the fascia and directed toward the pelvis (Fig. 3-4). To ensure that the insufflation needle is in the peritoneum, air is aspirated, a few milliliters of saline solution is injected through the needle (it should flow without resistance), the syringe is removed, and the column of saline solution is observed falling through the needle.

The needle is then connected to the insufflator and carbon dioxide is set to an initial flow of 1 to 4 L/min (Fig. 3-5). The diameter of the Veress needle precludes flow rates greater than 2.7 L/min. Once flow is established, the insufflator tubing is connected to a 10 mm sheath and the rate is increased to 4 to 5 L/min. The initial pressure during insufflation should be 4 to 6 mm Hg and certainly less than 10 mm Hg. This pressure level implies that there is free flow into the peritoneum without resistance and the needle is placed correctly. There have been some questions about the necessity for high-flow insufflators, which have recently been introduced. Because insufflation through the Veress needle is accomplished with a maximal flow rate of 2.7 L/min, there is little need for 8 to 10 L/min if the port resistance does not allow flow to approach this rate. Even with the larger 10 mm sheaths, flow rarely exceeds 5 L/min. My practice is to set the flow rate at 5 L/min and not alter it during the operation.

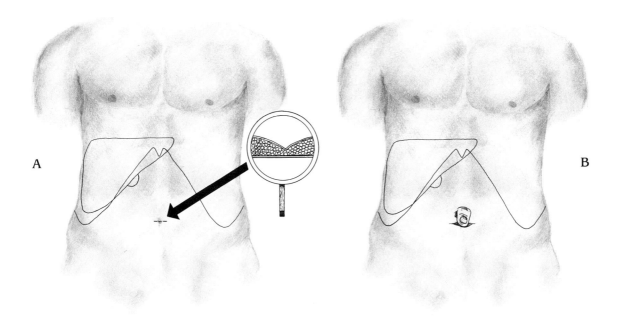

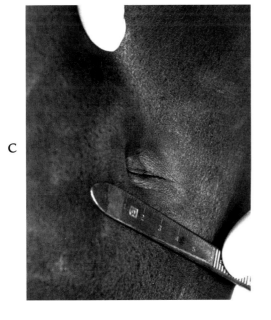

FIGURE 3-2 • **A,** A 1 cm transverse incision is made through the umbilicus. **B,** The subcutaneous tissue is bluntly dissected to the fascia with one's finger or knife handle. **C,** The length of the incision should be sufficient so that sheath of the port fits without force.

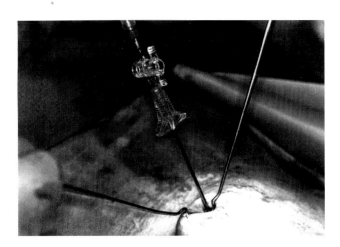

FIGURE 3-3 • In a thin patient, skin hooks may be used to elevate the fascia before placing the Veress needle. This maneuver may reduce the chance of retroperitoneal injury. It is more precise than lifting the skin of the abdominal wall.

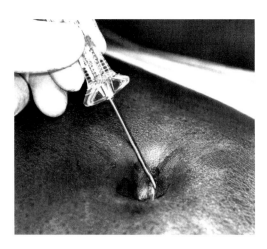

FIGURE 3-4 • The Veress needle is directed through the skin toward the pelvis.

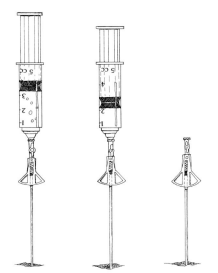

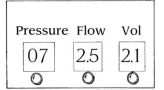

Pressure	Flow	Vol
07	2.5	2.1

FIGURE 3-5 • The position of the Veress needle in the peritoneal cavity is checked by several maneuvers. Air is aspirated from the peritoneal cavity, saline solution is injected, and the column of saline solution is observed falling into the abdominal cavity. When insufflation is begun, the pressure should be low (less than 8 mm Hg) with a flow rate between 1 and 2.7 L/min.

There is nothing sacred or fixed about umbilical placement of the camera port or establishment of insufflation by the Veress needle at the umbilicus. If the liver is enlarged, there may be little room to manipulate the camera if it is placed at the umbilicus. In this case, the camera should be repositioned beneath the umbilicus in the midline (Fig. 3-6, A).

If multiple adhesions or scars are present in the periumbilical region, the insufflation needle should be placed above the umbilicus or in the right upper quadrant (Fig. 3-6, B). These alternative sites are infrequently required but are very effective. In some instances the Veress needle will not enter the peritoneal cavity easily. This is a warning that should be heeded. The needle should not be forced because adhesions are probably present. The fascia should be opened and the underlying peritoneum explored digitally or by

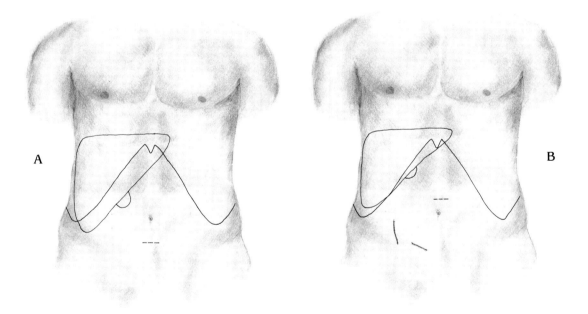

A   B

FIGURE 3-6 • **A,** When the liver is enlarged, camera mobility is reduced if placed through the umbilical port. Inserting the camera through an infraumbilical incision provides extra space and makes slippage of the port less likely. **B,** Previous abdominal surgery and hepatomegaly may preclude umbilical placement. In this situation the port can be placed above the umbilicus.

instrument (Fig. 3-7, *A*). The adhesions should be freed and the abdominal cavity beneath the fascia visualized. To do this, the trocar must be removed from the 10 mm port and either the sheath of the port must be placed into the abdomen or a special open laparoscopic port must be used (Fig. 3-7, *B*). A seal around this port should be made with sutures or towel clips and insufflation should be initiated at 4 to 6 L/min. An alternative is to use a port specifically designed for open laparoscopy (Fig. 3-7, *C*). It has a short sheath, a beveled hub (to hold it in the fascia), and wings that are sutured to the fascia to maintain its position. Although open laparoscopy is always an alternative, adhesions in the umbilical area may make port placement difficult even with the open technique. If this is the case, placement of the Veress needle in the right upper quadrant should be reconsidered. Another possible technique is to perform an initial direct placement of a 10 mm sheathed trocar into the abdomen. This technique must be done by experienced laparoscopists

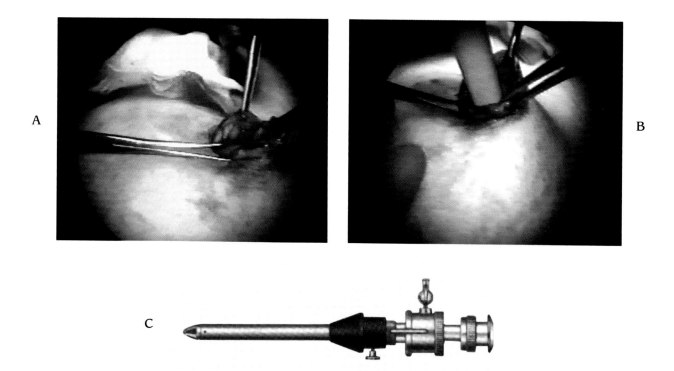

FIGURE 3-7 • **A,** This patient had an umbilical hernia. Once the 1 cm transverse incision was made in the umbilicus, preperitoneal fat was reduced and the incision in the fascia was cleared so that direct open laparoscopy could be done. **B,** A 10 mm sheath was introduced (without its trocar) into the peritoneal cavity. Towel clips were placed around it to prevent air leak. **C,** Cannula for establishing pneumoperitoneum without Veress needle or sharp trocar.

because it involves an increased risk of injury. I have no experience with this technique.

Once full pneumoperitoneum is achieved (pressure 15±3 mm Hg), the 10 mm port is slipped through the umbilicus, directed at a 45-degree angle toward the pelvis using steady and gentle pressure (Fig. 3-8). The distended abdomen makes it more difficult to penetrate the retroperitoneum. As soon as resistance lessens on the trocar, the trocar should be directed upward to the abdominal wall. These two maneuvers (gentle pressure into the peritoneum; upward direction once in the abdomen) limit pelvic injuries.

The scope is then inserted through the sheath in the umbilicus. Since operating rooms are cooler than the abdominal cavity, the scope will fog when placed in the abdomen. The easiest way to prevent this fogging is to immerse the scope in warm saline solution for 30 to 40 seconds before its use. This practice equilibrates the temperature of the scope with body temperature. During the operation, repeating this sequence or using an antifog solution helps to clear the lens. Touching the end of the laparoscope to the viscera also helps to keep the lens clear.

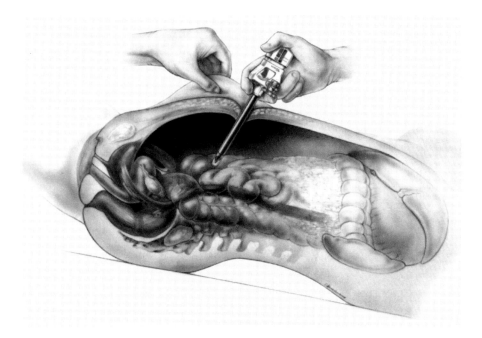

FIGURE 3-8 • Insertion of trocar and sheath, aimed at a 45-degree angle toward the pelvis. Lifting the skin, as shown here, often does just that, without elevating the fascia. A full pneumoperitoneum helps to cushion the entry force of the trocar and protect the bowel and retroperitoneal vessels.

As soon as the scope enters the sheath, the view at the bottom of the port should be clear (Fig. 3-9). When the scope is advanced, a complete examination is done of all pelvic and intra-abdominal viscera, and coexistent pathologic conditions are sought (Fig. 3-10). The right lower quadrant is examined to ascertain if it is adhesion free. This site is the entry point for the 5 mm ports. The table is then tilted (head up) at least 20 to 30 degrees (Fig. 3-11). This repositioning separates the transverse colon from the liver and

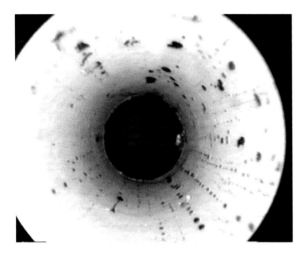

FIGURE 3-9 • When the camera and laparoscope are first introduced into the shaft of the 10 mm port, the view at the bottom should be clear. If it is cloudy, withdraw the scope and clean the lens.

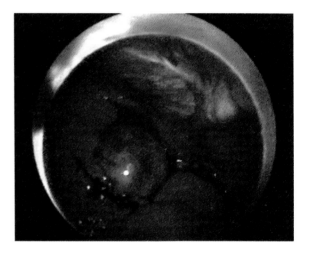

FIGURE 3-10 • The importance of a complete and thorough laparoscopic examination is evidenced with this patient. A large hemorrhagic corpus luteum cyst was found. It was aspirated and biopsied at the completion of the cholecystectomy.

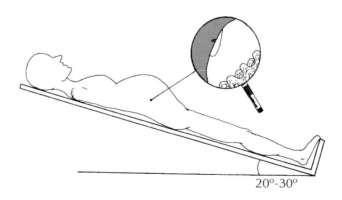

20°-30°

FIGURE 3-11 • The table is tilted 20 to 30 degrees. This maneuver further separates the transverse colon from the liver (inset).

gallbladder and exposes the gallbladder fundus. If the duodenum obscures the view of the lower part of the gallbladder, the operating table should be rotated 15 degrees to the left.

The placement of the 5 mm ports for instrumentation access to manipulate the gallbladder is relatively simple. Incorrect placement (usually too close to the ribs) is the reason sheaths slip and retract onto the abdominal wall during instrument transfer, resulting in gas leaks. Too often the ports are placed too close to the gallbladder and there is insufficient room between the end of the sheath and the gallbladder to manipulate instruments. Ports should be placed *at least one to one and one-half port lengths* from the gallbladder so that grasping and dissecting instruments can function effectively without the surgeon having to reposition or resecure the ports (Fig. 3-12). Once placed, ports should serve as fixed conduits.

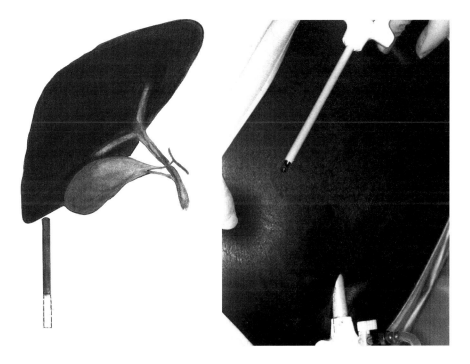

FIGURE 3-12 • By marking the position of the gallbladder (sighted by video) with one's finger, measuring one to one and one-half sheath lengths of a port, and inserting the port at that point, the surgeon allows sufficient distance between the end of the sheath and the gallbladder so that instruments can be maneuvered without having to retract and readjust the sheath.

Instruments placed through the lateral or fundic port are used to manipulate and secure the upper half of the gallbladder (Fig. 3-13). The port should not be placed in the subcostal position. It is preferably placed in the axis of the anterior axillary line just above the anterior superior iliac spine, but its position depends on the gallbladder location. If the fundic port is placed lateral to the anterior axillary line, instruments may get caught in the gutter of the right colon. I advise tracking the port with the camera as it enters the abdomen, but if the lower quadrant is free of adhesions, it is not necessary. The cushion of gas between the abdominal wall and bowel prevents injury, particularly when the port is directed toward the gallbladder. With the patient in the reverse Trendelenburg position, the sheath will maintain its position

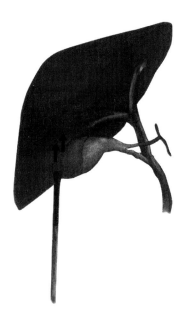

FIGURE 3-13 • Instruments placed through the fundic port are used to control the upper to middle portion of the gallbladder. This port is the first placed. It is positioned in the anterior axillary line so that there is enough distance between the end of the sheath and the gallbladder for instruments to function. The clamp placed through this port is used to expose the upper half of the gallbladder.

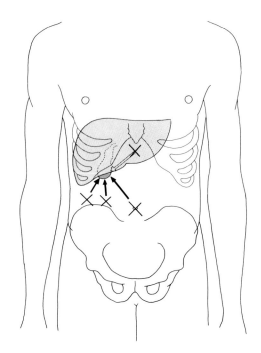

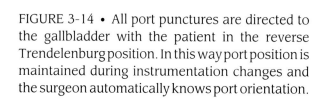

FIGURE 3-14 • All port punctures are directed to the gallbladder with the patient in the reverse Trendelenburg position. In this way port position is maintained during instrumentation changes and the surgeon automatically knows port orientation.

toward the gallbladder when instruments are removed, making repositioning of and searching for the port and instrument unnecessary. By directing *all*
ports to the gallbladder, one then intuitively knows where instruments are
relative to the scope, which saves considerable time and frustration (Fig. 3-
14).

A ratchet clamp is utilized to grasp the fundus of the gallbladder and push it
up to the diaphragm. This elevates the gallbladder out of its fossa and exposes
the lower portion of gallbladder. The infundibular port is then placed near but
above and medial to the fundic port. It will not interfere with the operation
of the laparoscope in this position, and placing it lateral to the rectus muscle
avoids injury to the epigastric vessels. Instruments through this port are used
to control the infundibulum of the gallbladder and expose the cystic duct and
cystic artery through upward, pelvic, and lateral traction (Fig. 3-15).

Placement of the 10 mm operating or upper midline port is critical as the
operating instruments should be visualized in front of or at right angles to the
laparoscope (Fig. 3-16). One common mistake is to insert this port too low in
the upper abdomen. Here, it will get in the way of the laparoscope or the scope
will block the view of the instruments. For this reason the operating port is

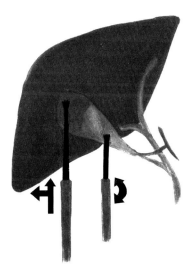

FIGURE 3-15 • Instruments placed through the infundibular port are used to control
the cystic duct and lower portions of the gallbladder. This port is placed superior and
medial to the fundic port. The arrows indicate the direction of traction during most
operations.

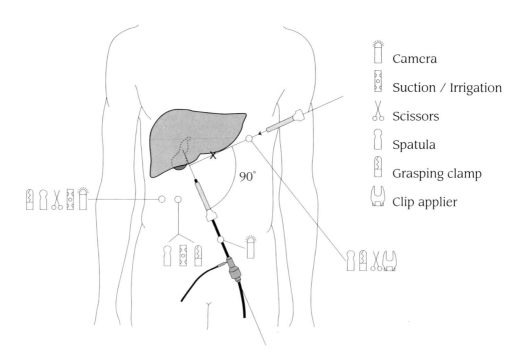

FIGURE 3-16 • Flexibility extends to instrument uses. Instrument placement depends on each anatomic situation. The key indicates multiuses of each port.

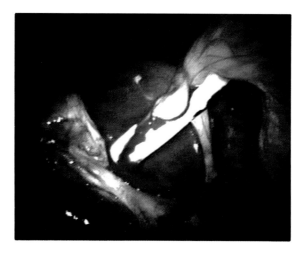

FIGURE 3-17 • The operating port can be placed on either side of the falciform ligament but not through it. As can be seen in this view, the operating port placed through the falciform ligament caused bleeding from the ligament. A clear view of the cystic artery and cystic duct was obtained, and tenting of the common duct was observed. Although the bleeding is rarely serious, it can obscure the operative field for several minutes until it stops spontaneously. Placing the port puncture too far to the right of the midline can cause bleeding from the epigastric vessels.

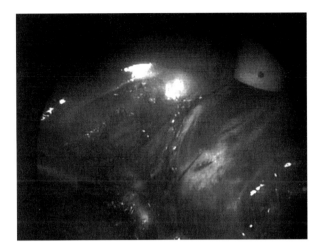

FIGURE 3-18 • The operating port placed high in the epigastrium serves as a useful retractor for the left lobe of the liver, which is an added advantage of this placement.

placed high in the abdomen, usually just beneath the xiphoid and to the right of the falciform ligament, which avoids bleeding from the falciform ligament near the costal margin (Fig. 3-17). If the falciform ligament is thin, another placement is to position the port to the left of the midline with the sheath advanced beneath the falciform ligament. The sheath of the 10 mm port is directed to the infundibulum of the gallbladder and may be used to retract a floppy left lobe of the liver (Fig. 3-18). I often use the sheath of the operating port to free omental adhesions from the infundibular portion of the gallbladder. This blunt dissection is safe and avoids injury to any structures.

Insufflation achieved and ports appropriately placed, cholecystectomy can proceed.

REFERENCE

1. Tompkins R. Laparoscopic cholecystectomy: Threat or opportunity? Arch Surg 125:1245, 1990.

·4·

Basic Operative Steps

Preview

- Few instrument transfers and application of appropriate traction and countertraction facilitate the operation.
- The areolar tissue and peritoneum over the cystic duct are incised with a cautery, and the spatula is moved in an up-and-down sweeping motion parallel to the cystic duct to free the duct.
- The cystic duct–common duct junction and the hepatic duct coursing to the liver must be visualized.
- Repositioning the grasping clamps facilitates removal of the gallbladder from the liver bed.
- Removing the gallbladder through the operating port is simple and avoids having to reposition the camera and instruments.

Laparoscopic cholecystectomy is ideal for the treatment of chronic cholecystitis. A normal thin-walled gallbladder can be easily manipulated with the laparoscopic instruments presently available, and the close-up exposure laparoscopy offers is accurate and clear. The procedure is simplified by using few instruments and maintaining constant traction on the gallbladder throughout the procedure and during instrument changes.

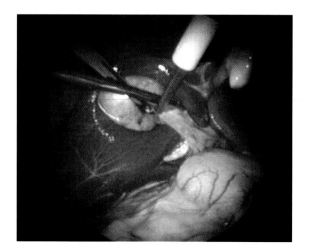

FIGURE 4-1 • Proper placement of clamps should lift the gallbladder and the undersurface of the liver and expose the hilar area. Stabilizing the gallbladder with an instrument placed in the operating port allows for easier repositioning of the gallbladder clamps.

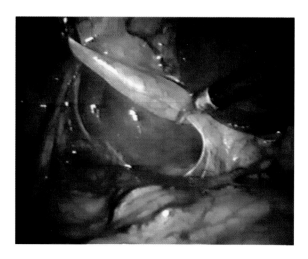

FIGURE 4-2 • The spatulated cautery was used to incise the peritoneum over the cystic duct.

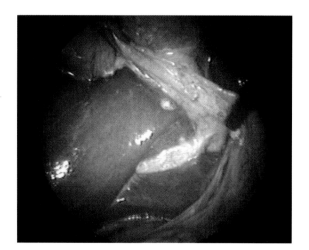

FIGURE 4-3 • With upward traction provided by the infundibular port clamp, the peritoneum near the cystic duct was swept toward the common duct.

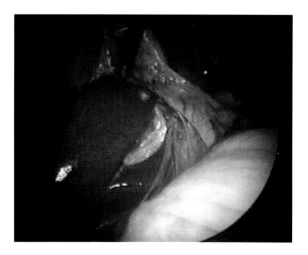

FIGURE 4-4 • The cystic duct, common duct, and common hepatic duct can be seen.

DISSECTION

For nearly all cases of chronic cholecystitis, appropriate traction on the gallbladder elevates it for proper viewing and dissection (Fig. 4-1). I use a spatula with an attached cautery and an air vent as the *only* dissecting instrument (Fig. 4-2). The cautery current is used to free adhesions and areolar tissue around the cystic duct; a sweeping upward and downward movement parallel to the cystic duct helps to free it (Fig. 4-3). The cystic duct–common duct junction must always be visualized, as should the exit of cystic duct from the gallbladder (Fig. 4-4). By passing the spatula up and down the cystic duct, the surgeon can feel and locate the cystic duct–common duct junction.

It is uncommon to visualize the upper hepatic duct with the camera positioned at the umbilicus. With the camera in this port, there is limited depth perception above the cystic duct, and the common duct appears distorted by traction placed on the infundibulum and cystic duct. If the cystic duct–common duct junction is not seen clearly, the infundibular port clamp can be placed on the cystic duct and upward traction applied. This maneuver may expose the common hepatic duct and facilitate dissection. If this approach fails, an angled viewing laparoscope should be used if available. If this type of laparoscope is not available or if visualization of the cystic duct–common duct junction with this scope is unsuccessful, the fundic 5 mm port should be replaced with a 10 mm port and the laparoscope inserted here (Fig. 4-5). With

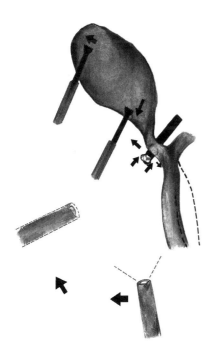

FIGURE 4-5 • Moving the laparoscope from the umbilical port to the fundic port (by replacing the 5 mm sheath with a 10 mm sheath) provides a more familiar view of the cystic duct–common duct junction.

the camera in this port, the common hepatic duct can almost always be seen above the cystic duct. This camera repositioning simulates the more familiar view available with open cholecystectomy since the surgeon's eye is parallel to the common duct and perpendicular to the cystic duct.

As an extra precaution, an operative cholangiogram taken through the gallbladder or cystic duct to display the duct anatomy may be helpful. The cholangiogram complements dissection and exposure but is not a substitute for visualization of the ducts.

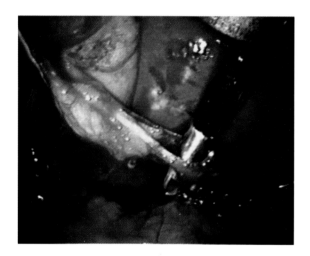

FIGURE 4-6 • Traction on the infundibulum of the gallbladder helps to create an avascular plane for dissection of the cystic artery. The cystic artery is shown with an instrument passed behind it. The clipped cystic duct is seen beneath the instrument tip.

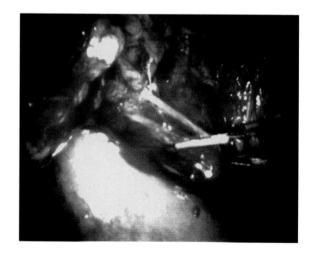

FIGURE 4-7 • A small posterior divisional branch of the cystic artery was encountered and clipped. Note the size difference between the 9 mm clip and the vessel.

SECURING THE CYSTIC ARTERY AND CYSTIC DUCT

Once the cystic duct–common duct junction is identified and its location confirmed by direct vision or cholangiography, the cystic duct is clipped singly or doubly (depending on its length) and divided, thus opening the base of the cystic triangle.

After the cystic duct is divided, the cystic artery is exposed by applying upward traction on the infundibulum of the gallbladder and sweeping the loose areolar tissue upward around the base of the gallbladder with the spatula. The artery is exposed, dissected, and encircled with scissors or spatulated cautery (Fig. 4-6). It is then clipped and divided. If a single small cystic artery is seen, it is likely to be an anterior divisional branch; during dissection of the gallbladder from the liver bed, a larger posterior divisional branch should be sought. Anticipating its presence and being cautious during dissection will avoid its transection and unnecessary bleeding (Fig. 4-7).

FREEING THE GALLBLADDER

When the cystic artery is secured and divided, traction is placed on the infundibulum of the gallbladder and the gallbladder is teased away from the liver bed. The avascular interface can be peeled away quite easily by cauterizing the peritoneum and sweeping the gallbladder away from the liver bed with the spatulated cautery or laser (Fig. 4-8). Excess smoke during cauterization or laser use implies that (1) the liver is being cauterized or "lasered," (2) insufficient tension is being placed on the gallbladder, or (3) the wrong plane is being dissected. Should the gallbladder be entered inadvertently, the infundibular port clamp can be easily repositioned to occlude the hole. If the hole is large, an EndoLoop can be placed around the neck of the gallbladder above the perforation, cinched down, and used as a retractor by grasping the cut end.

The position of the grasping clamps should be changed as needed during gallbladder removal to provide the best exposure and to allow dissection of the gallbladder to continue in an avascular plane. Watching an assistant struggle to replace a slipped clamp, the teeth of which are often ill prepared for the task, is both time consuming and frustrating. This situation is best

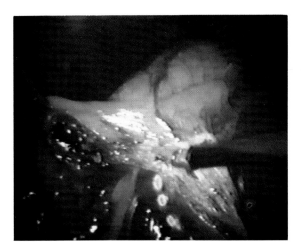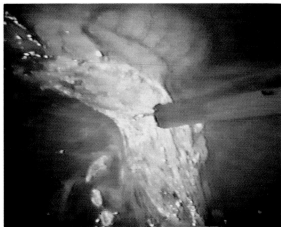

FIGURE 4-8 • Correct traction on the gallbladder allows the avascular plane between the gallbladder and the liver bed to be smoke-free during dissection. Changing the position of the infundibular port clamp as needed facilitates dissection.

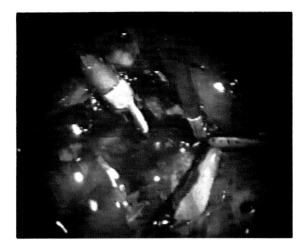

FIGURE 4-9 • The gallbladder bed is irrigated, cauterized, and retracted after the gallbladder is dissected from the liver. The gallbladder is then placed between the lateral abdominal wall and the liver. The simultaneous use of the suction/irrigator, spatula, and clamp allows exposure, irrigation, and cauterization in a clear field.

avoided by holding or stabilizing the gallbladder with an instrument placed through the operating port while the grasping clamp is repositioned. Countertraction is thus provided while the instrument is changed or secured.

Maintaining optimal exposure requires frequent instrument adjustments for floppy gallbladders and few adjustments for small gallbladders. If the gallbladder is deeply embedded or floppy, exposure of the posterior and inferior surfaces may be poor. In this situation the spatulated cautery should be moved to the infundibular port and a grasping clamp should be placed through the operating port. With the instruments in this position, the gallbladder and the inferior and medial surfaces of gallbladder peritoneum are exposed and splayed. With appropriate traction on the areolar tissue in the liver bed, the dissection proceeds smoothly. When traction on the gallbladder peritoneum is correct, the spatula should cut easily, that is, just touching the edge with the cautery should separate the gallbladder from the liver (Fig. 4-8). Freeing the gallbladder from the dome of liver is best done with scissors; repositioning the fundic port clamp onto the dome of the gallbladder close to the liver provides the needed tension for the cautery or laser to remain effective.

Once the gallbladder is separated completely from the liver bed, it is placed between the lateral abdominal wall and the liver. Clamps are removed from the gallbladder and are used to expose the gallbladder fossa. Irrigation and suction (through the operating port) and cauterization of small vessels and, rarely, an accessory bile duct (with a spatula in the infundibular port) are performed as needed before the gallbladder is removed (Fig. 4-9).

REMOVING THE GALLBLADDER

It is easier to remove the gallbladder through the operating port than to change the position of the laparoscope and remove the gallbladder through the umbilicus. Besides, if a thick-walled gallbladder slips from the clamp during its removal through the umbilicus, it may fall into the free peritoneal cavity below the transverse colon, where locating it can be fair game. Removing it through the operating port confines it to the area above the transverse colon.

From its position between the liver and abdominal wall, the gallbladder is grasped at its neck with a grasping clamp placed through the infundibular port, which stabilizes its position on the liver. A claw clamp (5 or 10 mm) placed through the operating port then is used to grasp the neck of the gallbladder near the cystic duct. The gallbladder is wedged into the sheath and the gallbladder and sheath are then withdrawn (Fig. 4-10). It is important to pull the neck of the gallbladder into the sheath. This action will ensure the delivery of the gallbladder onto the abdominal wall above the fascia as the sheath is withdrawn.

At times, difficulty in removing the gallbladder is encountered because of large stones. In this circumstance, the fascial opening must be enlarged by undermining the skin and extending the fascial incision. Decompressing the gallbladder will not facilitate delivery of a large stone or make a thick-walled gallbladder fit through a 1 cm fascial incision; the fascial incision must be extended.

Once the surgery is completed, the incisions are infiltrated with bupivacaine (Marcaine). Fascial incisions greater than 1 cm are closed with an absorbable suture. The other fascial puncture wounds are not sutured, but the subcuticular layer is approximated and a Band-Aid applied.

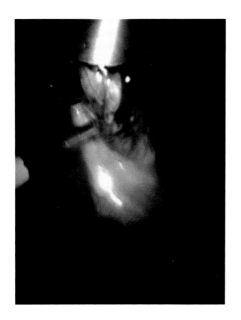

FIGURE 4-10 • The gallbladder was placed on the anterior surface of the liver to stabilize its position. It was then grasped near the cystic duct, withdrawn into the sheath of the operating port, and removed.

Illustrative Summary of Operative Technique

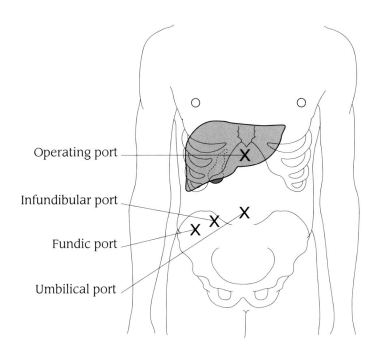

Although the placement of ports is individualized depending on gallbladder location, most surgeons position four ports. Some surgeons routinely place a fifth port; I use a fifth port only if the left lobe of the liver obscures the operative field or if better exposure is needed.

The 10 mm trocar is inserted through the umbilicus and is directed toward the pelvis, with little force exerted during its placement. The laparoscope and camera are then inserted through this port and used to thoroughly examine and explore the abdomen and pelvis.

The lateral or fundic port is placed next, usually at the anterior axillary line, at one to one and one-half port lengths below the gallbladder. Placement of the port at this location allows the instruments to function optimally without having to reposition the port. The infundibular port then is placed superior and 1 to 3 cm medial to the fundic port. This port position allows unrestricted movement and repositioning of clamps and provides ample room between the ports for instruments to manipulate the gallbladder. The operating port is placed high in the upper abdomen near the right xiphoid costal margin. This port allows instruments to operate in front of or at right angles to the laparoscope so they can be visualized throughout the procedure without having to reposition the camera. If the falciform ligament is thin, the port may be placed to its left. Keeping the port out of the falciform ligament avoids bleeding from the umbilical vein and facilitates removal of the gallbladder.

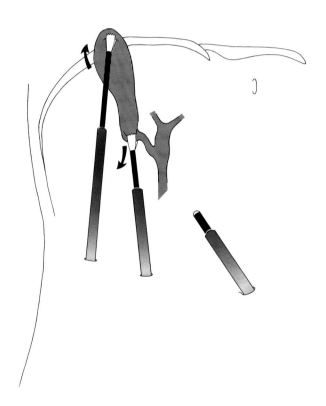

With upward traction on the fundus with the fundic port clamp and downward traction on the infundibulum with the infundibular port clamp (ratchet clamps preferred), the cystic duct is exposed. Repositioning the infundibular port clamp to the gallbladder–cystic duct junction improves cystic duct traction and exposure, particularly if the duct is elongated.

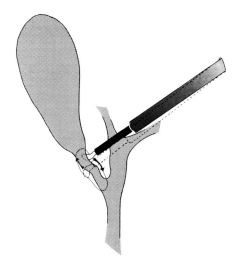

A cautery or laser current attached to a spatula is used to dissect the peritoneum around the duct, particularly at its inferior surface. The spatula is then used to free the cystic duct on all sides and is passed behind the duct, which helps to identify the cystic duct–common duct junction. The common duct *must* be visualized above and below the cystic duct. If the upper duct is not clearly seen, switching the camera to the fundic port may make it possible to visualize the upper duct.

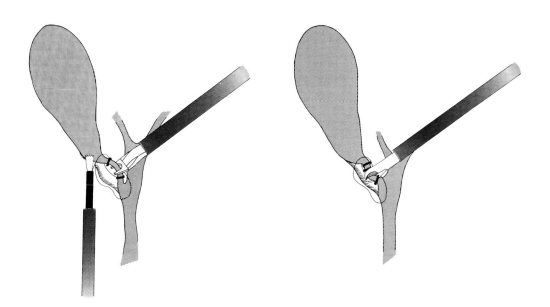

Continued traction on the infundibulum keeps the cystic duct taut and clips can be easily applied. With traction, two to four clips are applied to the cystic duct, depending on the length of the cystic duct and the surgeon's judgment. Before the cystic duct is transected, the common duct should again be identified above and below the cystic duct. Scissors, laser, or cautery can be used to divide the cystic duct. After the cystic duct is divided, the lumen should be totally occluded by the clip or tie.

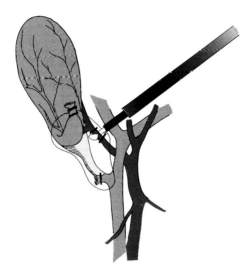

Upward traction on the infundibulum applied by pushing with the spatula or scissors will expose the cystic artery. The artery is looped with the spatula at its trunk or its divisional branches. If a small artery is encountered, a posterior divisional artery in the gallbladder fossa should be sought. The small artery can be controlled with cautery, laser, or clips.

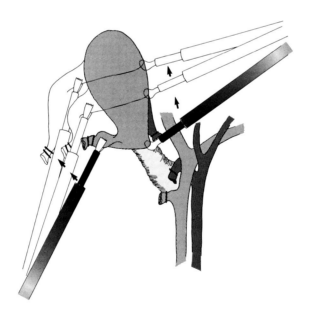

Continual repositioning of the infundibular port and fundic port clamps to maintain traction on the gallbladder and peritoneum is essential for optimal exposure and ease in freeing the gallbladder from the liver bed. When correct traction is applied, the laser or cautery will cause the gallbladder to peel away from the liver without creating smoke.

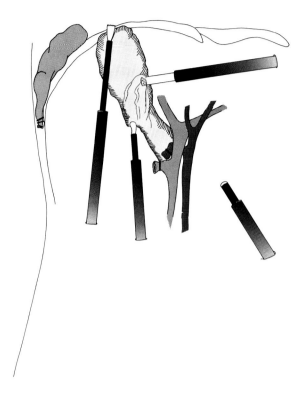

After the gallbladder is freed from the liver bed, it is placed between the liver and lateral abdominal wall. The clamps are released from the gallbladder and are used to expose the gallbladder fossa. The fossa is carefully examined for bleeding or a bile leak. If found, the sites are coagulated in the liver bed. Replacing the clamp in the infundibular port with the spatulated cautery allows exposure, irrigation, and coagulation of bleeding vessels to occur simultaneously.

Without the camera being repositioned, the gallbladder is grasped at its neck with a 5 mm or 10 mm clamp, pulled into the operating port sheath, and removed through the operating port. A drain may be placed through the fundic port if necessary.

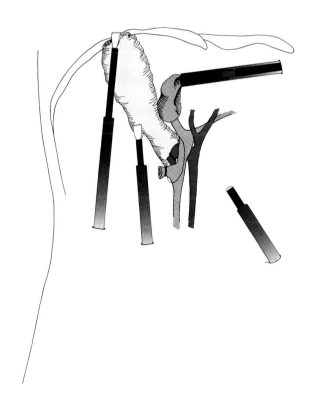

Case Presentations

Hilar Approach

CASE 1

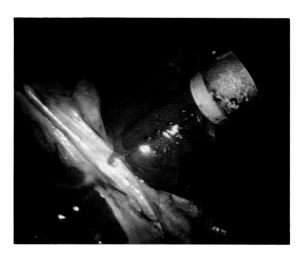

A 35-year-old woman underwent elective cholecystectomy for chronic recurrent cholecystitis. With proper upward traction on the infundibulum, the peritoneum over the cystic duct was stretched taut. The spatulated cautery was used to open the peritoneum and expose the cystic duct.

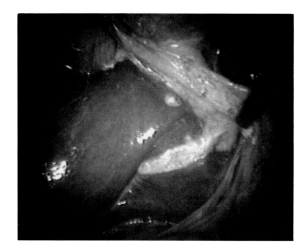

The peritoneum was incised, and an up-and-down motion with blunt dissection exposed the cystic duct. In this case, the cystic duct was small and could easily be encircled by the spatulated cautery. The shaft of the spatula was used to clear around the duct on all sides.

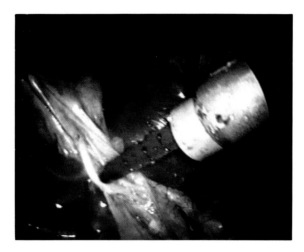

The common bile duct and the common hepatic duct were identified at the entrance of the cystic duct. The spatula is shown encircling the cystic duct. Clips were then placed across the cystic duct and it was transected.

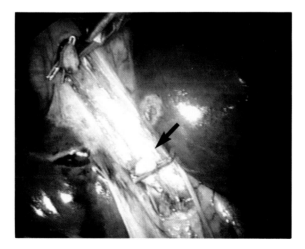

Upward traction with scissors on the peritoneum surrounding the cystic duct at the base of the gallbladder facilitated dissection and exposure of the cystic artery (arrow). The artery was exposed by sweeping the peritoneum upward. Clips were placed across the cystic artery and it was then transected.

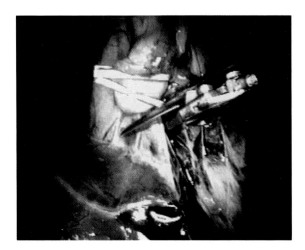

Scissors were used to transect and dissect the peritoneum at the lower end of the gallbladder. Appropriate traction with the infundibular port clamp exposed the peritoneum.

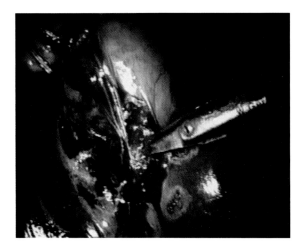

Scissors, connected to a cautery unit, provided effective control of bleeding in the liver bed. As in open cholecystectomy, scissors can be used to dissect the gallbladder.

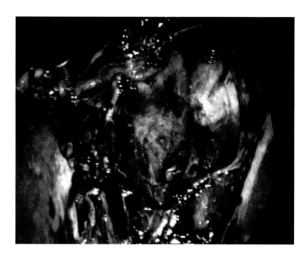

The gallbladder was dissected free of the liver bed and the peritoneal attachments at the dome of the gallbladder were exposed and transected with scissors.

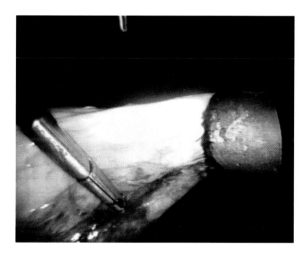

The gallbladder was placed in the operating port and easily withdrawn onto the abdominal wall.

Retrograde Approach

CASE 2

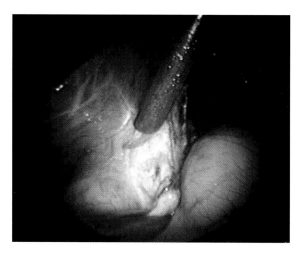

This 40-year-old woman with chronic cholecystitis and cholelithiasis underwent elective surgery. There was difficulty in dissecting the hilum and the lower third of the gallbladder. Accordingly, the fundus of the gallbladder was dissected from the liver bed with the spatulated cautery. A clamp from the operating port maintained upward traction on the liver, and downward traction on the gallbladder was provided by a clamp placed through the fundic port. The spatulated cautery was placed through the infundibular port.

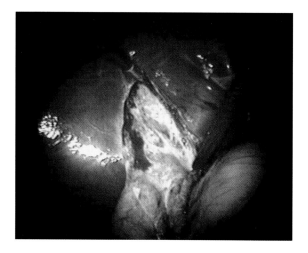

The gallbladder was peeled from the liver bed by applying downward traction on the gallbladder and upward countertraction on the liver. In this circumstance, a clamp from the fundic port maintained traction on the gallbladder, a clamp from the infundibular port maintained upward traction on the liver, and the spatula was placed through the operating port.

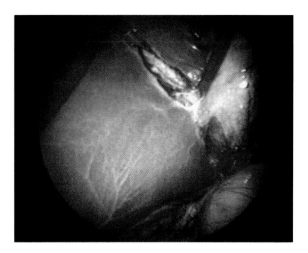

The peritoneum on the lower medial inferior third of the gallbladder was exposed and dissected. Clamps were repositioned so that suitable exposure and traction were maintained throughout the dissection.

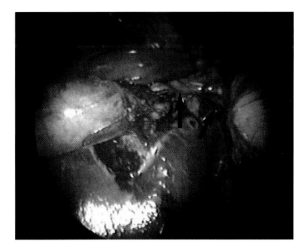

The gallbladder was completely dissected and freed from the liver bed. The cystic duct was seen with a convoluted spiral valve (left arrow). The common duct was located below it (right arrow).

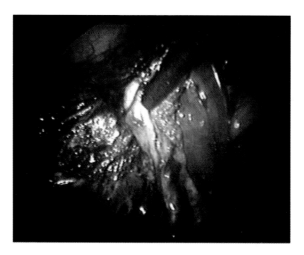

The spatula was placed around the circumference of the cystic duct, which was elongated. The cystic duct was triply clipped and divided between the two upper clips, completely freeing the gallbladder and cystic duct. The cystic duct–common duct junction could again be identified.

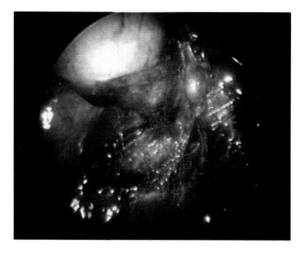

Scissors were used to transect the cystic duct. The cystic artery (upper arrow) was identified at its origin from the hepatic artery (lower arrow). It was dissected and encircled with the spatulated cautery.

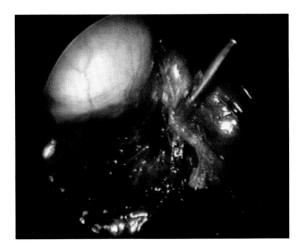

The cystic artery was clipped prior to its division. Because of the redundant length of the cystic duct, it was grasped and dissected closer to the common duct, where it was reclipped and transected.

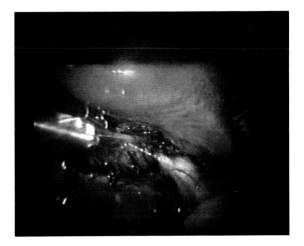

The area was irrigated through a suction/irrigation device placed through the infundibular port. The liver bed was retracted upward with a clamp placed through the operating port. The clip that was used to secure the cystic duct can be seen. The cystic duct, common duct, and hepatic duct are clearly visible.

Lateral Lower Third Approach

CASE 3

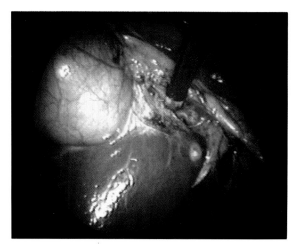

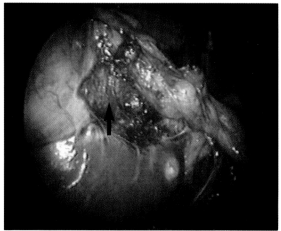
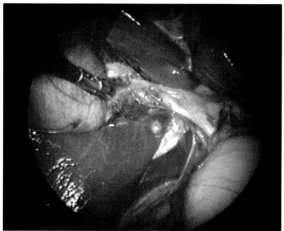

A 42-year-old woman with chronic cholecystitis underwent laparoscopic cholecystectomy. The peritoneum over the lower lateral third of the gallbladder was dissected to facilitate exposure and mobilization of the cystic duct. The lower common duct and the upper hepatic duct were not clearly identified through the hilar approach, despite freeing the peritoneum (arrow) on the inferior and superior surfaces of the cystic duct. This technique of freeing peritoneum inferiorly and superiorly at the lower third of the gallbladder often frees the cystic duct and the gallbladder, providing enough mobility so that the lower hepatic duct can then be identified. In this way the cystic duct is mobilized but not clipped until the end of the procedure, which ensures the integrity of the duct system.

·II·

Problems

·5·

The Difficult Cholecystectomy

Preview

- Empyema or hydrops of the gallbladder may require the use of a trocar to decompress and elevate the gallbladder.

- Retrograde, lower lateral third, or antegrade approaches may be needed to separate the gallbladder from the liver and expose the cystic duct and the common duct.

- Upward traction on the liver bed is provided by a clamp placed through the operating port. The spatula or scissors can be operated through the infundibular port or the fundic port.

- Once the common duct is identified above and below the cystic duct entry, the cystic duct and artery are isolated and clipped.

- A positional change of the camera to the fundic port may facilitate visualization of the common duct.

- Copious irrigation of the operative field may limit infections.

- Drains may be used as required.

———————

As experience and confidence with laparoscopic cholecystectomy increase, its applications will liberalize. The determination of which cholecystectomies can be guided by the laparoscope is solely dependent on the facility, expertise, and judgment of the individual surgeon, particularly in terms of how the anatomic findings relate to the cystic duct, common duct, and cystic artery. At present, in many hospitals, only patients with chronic cholecystitis and cholelithiasis undergo laparoscopic cholecystectomy. Patients with palpable, tender gallbladders; patients with thick-walled, contracted, embedded gallbladders; or patients with suspected empyema or acute cholecystitis are refused laparoscopic cholecystectomy. This selection is based on an unsubstantiated fear that the intraoperative technical difficulties will preclude a satisfactory outcome. The frequency of patients presenting with gallbladders deemed "difficult" varies among hospitals and with each surgeon's referral practice. Their number seems to increase directly and proportionately with one's experience! Removal of these problem gallbladders is not as difficult as feared, and their presence certainly should not be a contraindication to laparoscopic cholecystectomy. Patients with such gallbladders presently constitute 30% to 40% of the cholecystectomy patients I treat.

From the outset, it should be kept in mind that operative findings are unpredictable. Some patients with a paucity of symptoms have chronically contracted or embedded gallbladders with obstructed cystic ducts, whereas others with acute symptoms have no adhesions and an easily dissectable gallbladder. Because of these unpredictable findings, I laparoscopically examine the gallbladder in every case of acute and chronic cholecystitis to try to ascertain the degree of difficulty I can expect to encounter in its removal. There need be no arbitrary exclusions. Almost all gallbladders are suitable for laparoscopic surgery. As a general rule, if the gallbladder can be seen with the laparoscope, it can be safely removed.

OPERATIVE STRATEGIES

The operative strategy for removing the difficult gallbladder requires much more flexibility than that for removing the gallbladder in chronic cholecystitis because the surgeon must be willing to improvise and to do the operation antegrade or retrograde. With a difficult inflamed gallbladder, the greater omentum frequently encases and surrounds the gallbladder, which obscures the view of the gallbladder. The omentum must first be retracted and freed with grasping forceps, scissors attached to a cautery unit, or spatulated cautery. The omentum usually peels off fairly easily. If the gallbladder is distended, an attempt is made to decompress it with a trocar. Since the lumen of the trocar needle is small, it is only effective for aspirating thin, watery bile; thick, purulent bile cannot be aspirated with the trocar needle (Fig. 5-1).

If possible, dissection should begin at the infundibulum of the gallbladder. Clamps are placed in the usual position, but if the clamps cannot maintain traction, they are removed and a long aspirating trocar is placed into the lower part of the gallbladder and used as a lifting retractor (Fig. 5-2). At times, I cauterize a hole in the dome of the gallbladder and then empty it with a large (10 mm) suction device. Spilled stones that invariably accompany this maneuver can be retrieved individually, placed into a stone bag, or replaced in the gallbladder at the end of the procedure. The emptied gallbladder is easier to grasp.

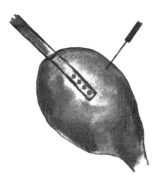

FIGURE 5-1 • Emptying the gallbladder can be more difficult at laparoscopy than at open surgery. The small trocar needle has a diameter that is too small to aspirate anything but watery bile. When there is thick purulent material, a hole can be cauterized in the fundus of the gallbladder and a larger bore trocar or chest tube inserted to decompress the gallbladder.

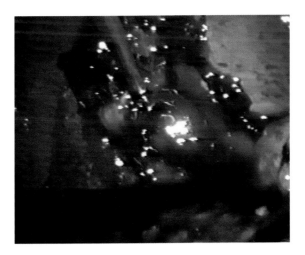

FIGURE 5-2 • A clamp proved ineffective in maintaining traction on the gallbladder. A trocar was introduced to elevate the gallbladder out of its fossa.

With the same technique as that used for gallbladder removal in chronic cholecystitis, the cystic artery and cystic duct are isolated in the hilum. Since the cystic duct is usually encountered first, the peritoneum and areolar tissue over the infundibulum of the gallbladder and upper cystic duct are cauterized and dissected. Often this process is tedious, and the inflamed edematous tissue obscures the hilar anatomy, making this approach unsafe or too difficult. In this case, the gallbladder is rotated medially and laterally so the peritoneal interface between the lower one third of the gallbladder and the liver bed is freed. This maneuver, particularly the inferior dissection, is facilitated by placing the spatula in the infundibular port (Fig. 5-3). A grasper placed in the operating port splays the gallbladder. Sometimes mobilizing the lower third of the gallbladder at the liver junction will free the cystic duct and allow the duct to be accurately isolated near the gallbladder. It can then be encircled from behind.

If this approach cannot be done because the gallbladder is embedded in the liver or is severely inflamed, the gallbladder should be dissected retrograde. Traction is placed on the fundus with grasping forceps. The infundibular port

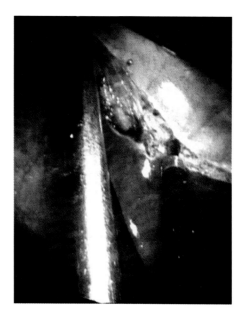

FIGURE 5-3 • The lower peritoneum was dissected with the spatulated cautery placed through the infundibular port. Traction by clamps placed through the operating port and the fundic port splayed the gallbladder.

clamp is placed between the fundus of gallbladder and the liver and used to push the liver from gallbladder (Fig. 5-4). The peritoneum over the gallbladder, which in the case of an inflamed gallbladder consists of a thick fibrinous peel, is dissected between the liver and gallbladder using the spatulated cautery or scissors. The avascular plane is difficult to locate and may seem nonexistent, but once entered, the magnified view on the monitor facilitates dissection (Fig. 5-5). Once the peritoneum is dissected, the gallbladder wall can be seen. The gallbladder wall itself is not as thick as the peel and it can be grasped with a clamp. Dissection continues from the fundus downward so that the upper and lateral portions of the gallbladder are freed completely from the liver. In some cases adhesions between the gallbladder and liver can

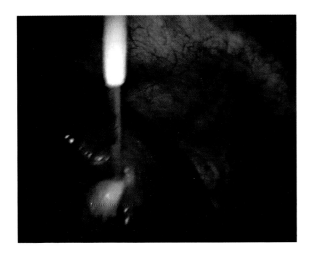

FIGURE 5-4 • The gallbladder was grasped at its fundus and the liver retracted with a long clamp placed through the operating port.

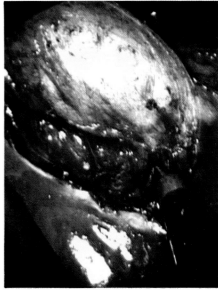

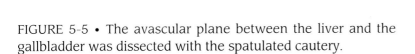

FIGURE 5-5 • The avascular plane between the liver and the gallbladder was dissected with the spatulated cautery.

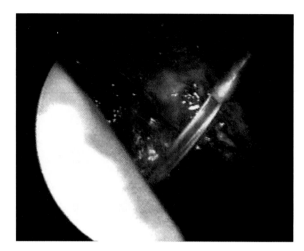

FIGURE 5-6 • Hydrodissection may facilitate blunt dissection of gangrenous and embedded gallbladders. The flow of saline solution maintains good vision in the area, and the metal tip of the suction/irrigation probe acts as a good blunt dissecting instrument.

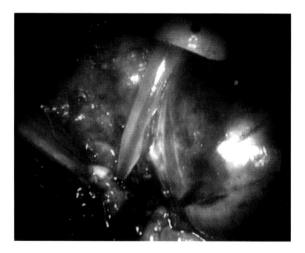

FIGURE 5-7 • The cystic duct diameter exceeded that with which I am comfortable for application of clips. Therefore, after the gallbladder was transected, an EndoLoop inserted through the operating port was placed around the cystic duct by placing the grasping forceps through the EndoLoop and then pushing the knot down onto the cystic duct.

be so dense that the spatulated cautery is ineffective. A hydrodissector (a blunt suction/irrigation tip) or scissors are used to free the gallbladder from the liver bed (Fig. 5-6). As the lower third of the gallbladder is approached, the posterior branch of the cystic artery must be sought. Once identified, it is clipped. If the artery is accidentally transected, it must be compressed to control bleeding and then clipped or coagulated.

The last structure to be isolated is the cystic duct. The cystic duct should be traced to its entry into the common duct, and the common duct above and below the cystic duct should be accurately identified. If the cystic duct is thick walled, it should be encircled with an EndoLoop, which is cinched down. The duct is transected above the knot. Alternatively, the duct may be transected first and then the EndoLoop placed and tied (Fig. 5-7).

In difficult cholecystectomies, spillage of bile often occurs from trauma caused by clamping, from entrance of incorrect planes of dissection, or from perforation of the gallbladder. When bile is spilled, the bed of the liver must be copiously lavaged to prevent subhepatic infection. In three of the first 30 operations I performed on patients with difficult gallbladders, subhepatic collections developed postoperatively because of contamination of an incompletely evacuated hematoma in the subhepatic space. With the use of a stronger pressure for irrigation, I have found that the subhepatic space is now more effectively cleared (Fig. 5-8). Since the practice of using higher pressure with the irrigation system was instituted, I have not had this problem.

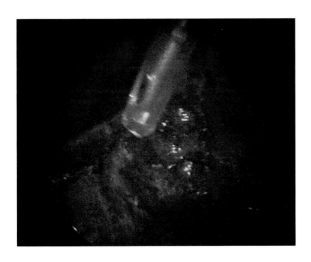

FIGURE 5-8 • The gallbladder was freed and placed between the lateral abdominal wall and liver. The gallbladder fossa was irrigated with saline solution and suctioned.

DRAINING THE SUBHEPATIC SPACE

If the gallbladder dissection has been difficult or if there has been oozing in the liver bed, the surgeon may wish to drain the gallbladder fossa. Inserting a drain into the subhepatic space is a relatively simple procedure that may help to safeguard against infection.

To insert the drain, the fundic port is removed and the puncture site is covered. The end of a 7 to 10 mm soft vinyl Jackson-Pratt drain is clamped with a long clamp to prevent gas leak, and the drain is shortened (by cutting 3 inches off the end) and is pushed with a needle holder through the lateral puncture site into the peritoneal cavity. The drain is then grasped by a clamp placed through the operating port or the infundibular port (Fig. 5-9) and is positioned between the liver and the abdominal wall in the subhepatic space. It is connected briefly to suction to be certain it is positioned effectively and then reclamped so that pneumoperitoneum is not lost. A recently described clever method of inserting the drain is to place a long clamp from the fundic port through the operating port to the abdominal wall, where it is used to grasp and then pull the drain into the abdomen (personal communication, John A. Dutro, M.D., August 1991) (Fig. 5-10).

The use of drains is reassuring and helpful. Depending on the nature and quantity of drainage postoperatively, the drain is left in place from 12 hours to several days. The patient is instructed about caring for the drain site.

POSTOPERATIVE CARE

Postoperative care is similar to that following open cholecystectomy for chronic cholecystitis. The patient is allowed a clear liquid diet several hours after surgery, which is advanced quickly to a regular diet, and antibiotic administration is continued for 5 to 7 days. This is an empiric judgment; the length of time and necessity for antibiotic administration have not been demonstrated. Patients are kept overnight and dismissed the following morning.

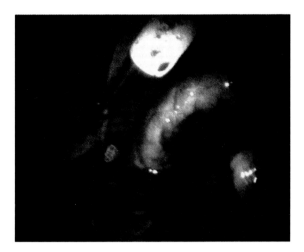

FIGURE 5-9 • Because the gallbladder had been deeply embedded and extensively gangrenous, a 10 mm Jackson-Pratt drain was introduced through the fundic port by removing the 5 mm port and occluding the puncture site with my finger. The drain was advanced on a needle holder into the peritoneal cavity through the puncture. A clamp placed through the operating port positioned the drain in the right lateral gutter and subhepatic space. Its position was verified by connecting it to suction.

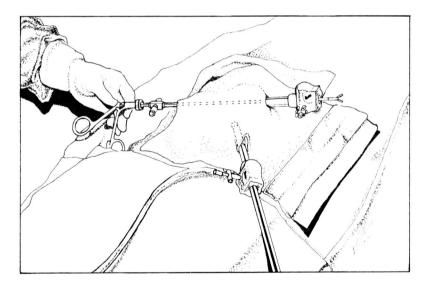

FIGURE 5-10 • An alternative method of drain placement has been suggested. A clamp from the fundic port is brought through the sheath of the operating port, and the drain is pulled into the abdomen and positioned. (Figure courtesy John A. Dutro, M.D., Dayton, Ohio.)

Illustrative Summary of Retrograde Cholecystectomy

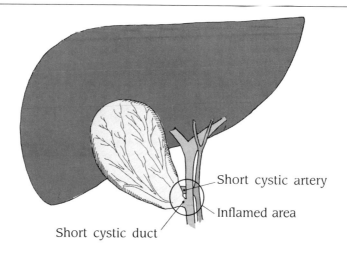

Short cystic artery

Inflamed area

Short cystic duct

If there is severe inflammation in the hilum, exposure and access to the hilar structures may be limited. It may not be possible to dissect the cystic duct and cystic artery antegrade.

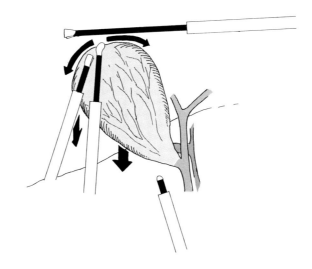

In this circumstance, the gallbladder fundus is grasped while the edge of the liver is pushed away from the gallbladder, providing countertraction. The spatula is introduced through the infundibular port or the fundic port, and the peritoneum at the dome of the gallbladder is incised. Downward traction on the gallbladder and upward pressure on the liver edge allow the gallbladder to be separated from the liver bed. A clamp placed through the operating port maintains uniform traction on the liver without entering or injuring it. If clamps do not hold, an aspirating trocar placed in the gallbladder lumen can be used to elevate the gallbladder.

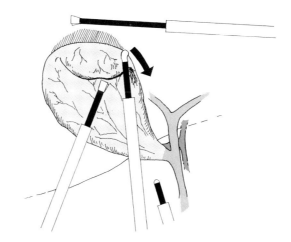

The fundus of the gallbladder is dissected free from the liver bed, which often entails entering a thick peel to expose the gallbladder. The dissection is carried on both sides of the gallbladder to its lower third. The grasping clamps are continually repositioned to provide suitable access and exposure.

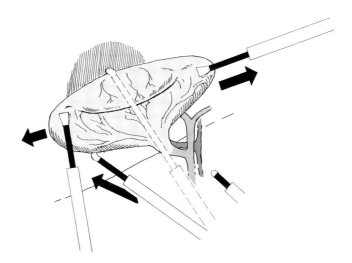

Continual traction and countertraction on the gallbladder and liver bed facilitate complete dissection. Constant reappraisal of optimal cautery or laser application must be done so that appropriate traction and exposure are maintained.

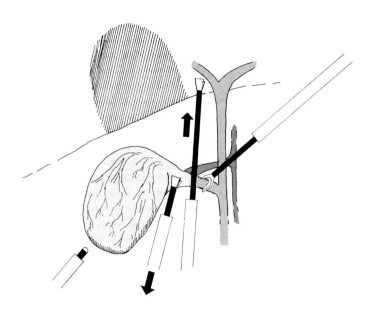

When the gallbladder is freed, the cystic duct–common duct junction should be seen clearly and the common duct must be identified above and below the cystic duct. If these structures cannot be accurately visualized, the fundic 5 mm port is replaced with a 10 mm port and the camera is repositioned here. From this perspective the common duct should be visible above the cystic duct. The clip applier is placed around the cystic duct. One set of grasping forceps is used to apply downward traction on the gallbladder while the other is used to push up on the liver. Excellent exposure and visualization of the cystic duct are thus obtained.

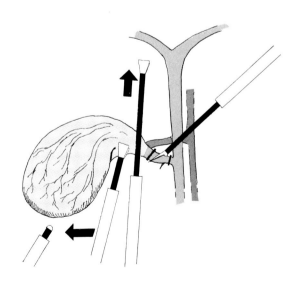

The cystic duct is then clipped and divided.

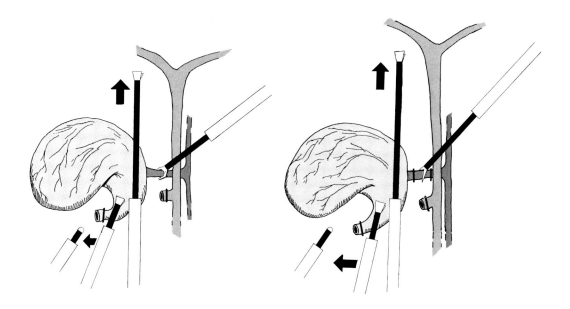

The cystic artery is isolated, clipped, and divided in a similar manner.

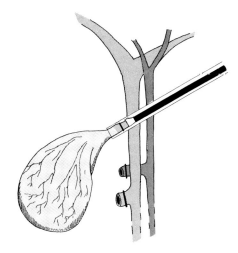

The gallbladder is removed through the operating port. A 10 mm Jackson-Pratt drain is usually placed through the fundic port to collect any oozing or bile leak.

Case Presentations

RETROGRADE DISSECTION

CASE 1

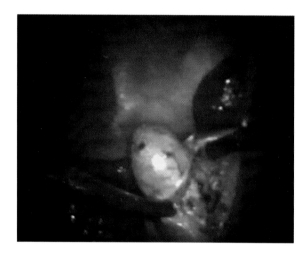

This deeply embedded, acutely distended gallbladder had a hilum that was obscured and difficult to dissect because of inflammation. The gallbladder was grasped at its middle to lateral body, and a clamp placed through the operating port retracted the undersurface of the liver. The avascular gall-bladder-peritoneum interface was thus exposed, allowing the lateral peritoneum to be dissected with the spatulated cautery placed through the infundibular port.

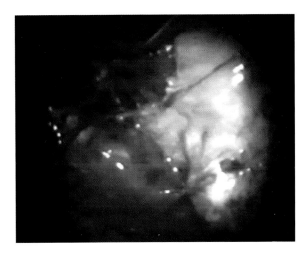

Dissection was carried medially to free the medial surface of the gallbladder. The clamps were repositioned so that the spatulated cautery could work effectively through the infundibular port while the fundic port clamp held the upper gallbladder. A clamp placed on the infundibulum of the gallbladder through the operating port splayed the gallbladder and exposed the peritoneum on the medial inferior surface.

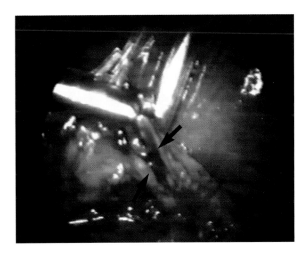

Retrograde dissection of the gallbladder was continued until the cystic duct (lower arrow) and cystic artery (upper arrow) were seen. The cystic duct was clearly identified separate from the common duct. Clamps were used to elevate the cystic artery, which was freed by blunt dissection.

ADHESIONS
Sharp Dissection

CASE 2

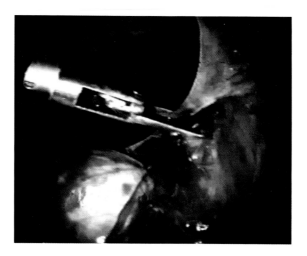

A patient who had undergone multiple previous abdominal operations had inflammatory adhesions around the gallbladder. Adhesions between the gallbladder and the dome of liver were lysed by sharp dissection using straight scissors placed through the fundic port. Traction was provided with a clamp through the operating port. This dissection exposed the gallbladder fundus.

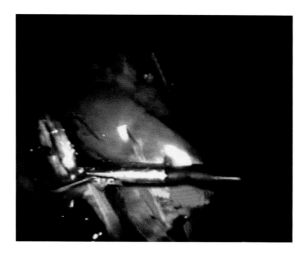

Scissor dissection effectively dissected the gallbladder from the liver bed.

Blunt Dissection

CASE 3

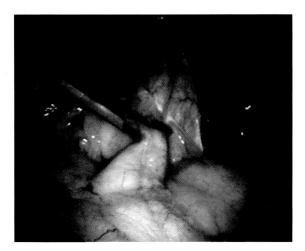

A 44-year-old man underwent elective cholecystectomy for recurrent chole-cystitis. The fundic port clamp was used to elevate the gallbladder and the infundibular port clamp was used to separate adhesions from the gallbladder by blunt dissection.

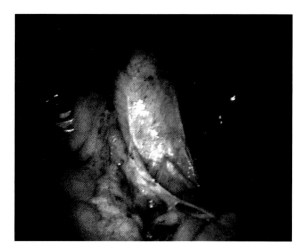

The gallbladder was freed from all adhesions and the infundibular port clamp was placed on the infundibular portion of the gallbladder.

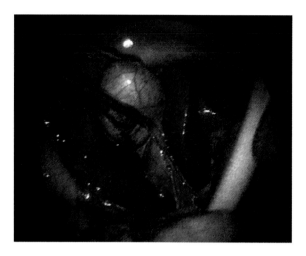

Upward traction was then placed on the gallbladder, and the operating port sheath was used to bluntly dissect adhesions between the lower infundibulum and the duodenum. The sheath of the trocar can be an effective blunt dissector for the infundibular portion of the gallbladder.

Cautery Dissection

CASE 4

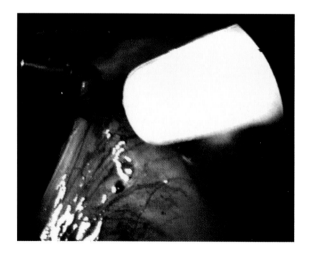

A patient with acute cholecystitis had thin adhesions between the gallbladder and omentum. With proper upward traction on the gallbladder, the spatulated cautery was used to dissect the vascular adhesions.

GANGRENOUS GALLBLADDER
Antegrade Approach

CASE 5

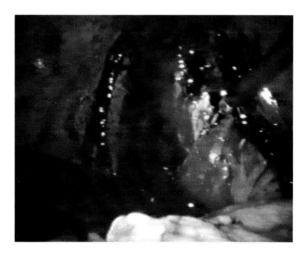

A patient who presented with minimal symptoms was found to have gangrenous cholecystitis. A thick peel surrounding the gallbladder made dissection difficult, but the peel was entered at the infundibular portion of the gallbladder. The spatulated cautery was used to dissect the peritoneum downward. Since clamps were ineffective in maintaining the position of the gallbladder, a trocar was used to stabilize the gallbladder and elevate it out of its fossa. The thick peel is seen to the lower right.

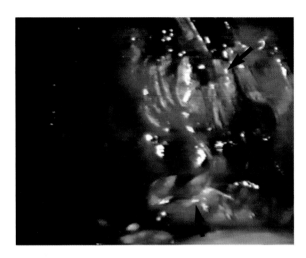

After the peel was freed, the infundibulum (upper arrow) was grasped with a clamp and elevated, which facilitated exposure of the cystic duct and cystic artery. It was noted that the cystic artery crossed the cystic duct. With the infundibulum elevated, the peel surrounding the gallbladder (lower arrow) was pushed away from the cystic duct.

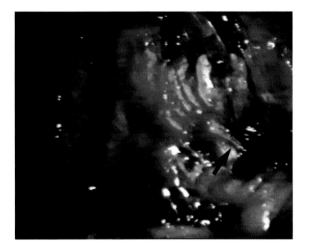

The cystic duct (lower arrow) and cystic artery (upper arrow) were divided between clips, and the gallbladder was dissected from the liver bed using a spatulated cautery and hydrodissector (a 5 mm suction/irrigation probe).

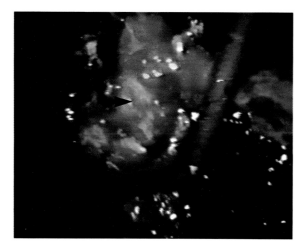

The gallbladder (arrow) was so gangrenous that it peeled away from the liver without resistance.

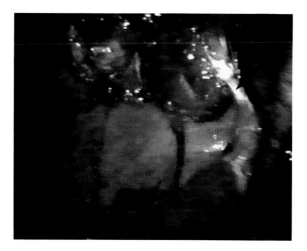

The gallbladder separated from the liver bed at its upper portion. The last attachment (arrow) was transected with scissors.

CASE 6

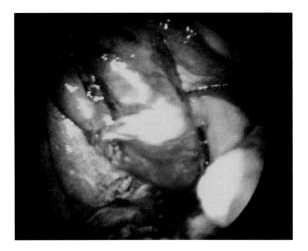

A gangrenous necrotic gallbladder was present in a 94-year-old man with mild symptoms. A trocar placed through the infundibular port was used to decompress and then elevate the gallbladder.

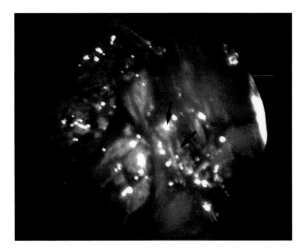

The cystic duct (lower arrow) was next exposed with the spatulated cautery. It was small and entered the common duct at a right angle. The gallbladder infundibulum is seen above (upper arrow).

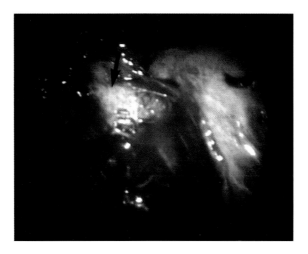

The gangrenous gallbladder (arrow) was dissected antegrade after the cystic artery and the cystic duct were ligated and divided. Because of the extensive amount of gangrene, dissection was not necessary: the traction clamps on the gallbladder literally pulled the gallbladder free from the liver bed.

Retrograde Approach: Situs Inversus

CASE 7

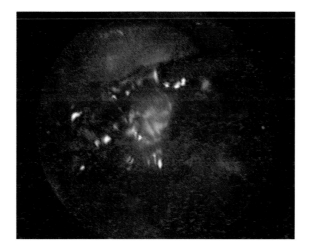

This 64-year-old woman presented with recurrent chronic and acute chole-cystitis and had an unrelenting attack that required hospitalization for 1 week. She had situs inversus as well. The gallbladder was exposed in the right upper quadrant after the transverse colon was dissected from the lateral and superior walls of the gallbladder.

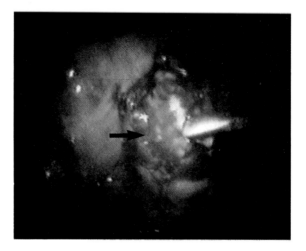

The gallbladder (arrow) was dissected from the liver with difficulty. A trocar was used to stabilize and maintain the position of the gallbladder since clamps proved ineffective in providing traction. Despite the gallbladder being emptied of bile, the wall was thickened and clamps were still ineffective for much of the procedure. The inflammatory adhesions were so dense that scissors were used.

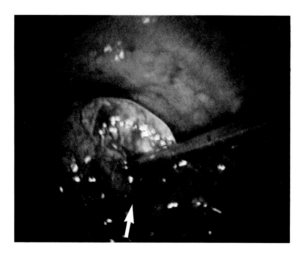

A small artery from the attached omentum was bleeding at the dome of the gallbladder (arrow). It was secured by clips.

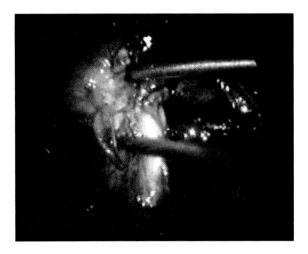

The trocar stabilized and maintained gallbladder position while the gallbladder was dissected from the liver bed. Another clamp was placed to provide additional traction.

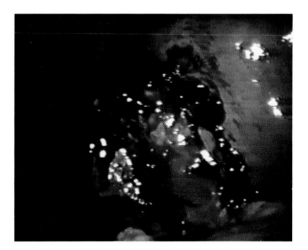

The exposed gangrenous gallbladder was dissected from the liver bed.

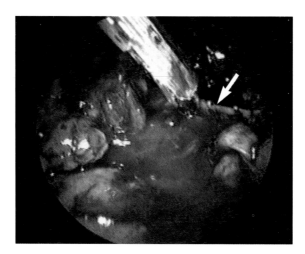

A posterior cystic artery (arrow) was identified, clipped, and divided between the liver bed and gallbladder.

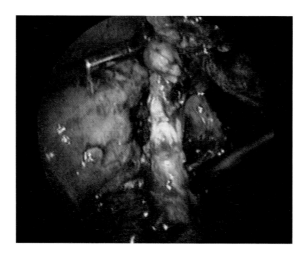

A large, elongated cystic duct was identified entering the common duct. A cholangiogram confirmed that no stones were present in the common duct. Because of the size of the cystic duct, an EndoLoop was placed to control it. A drain was placed after the gallbladder was removed.

• Invited Commentary •

Dr. Cooperman has extensive experience with the laparoscopic removal of the acutely inflamed gallbladder. The technique he describes of removing the gallbladder from the fundus toward the infundibulum is an unusual approach and offers a solution when severe inflammation renders initial dissection of Calot's triangle dangerous.

At Washington University in St. Louis we have encountered many patients with acutely inflamed or gangrenous gallbladders and have used many of the same techniques Dr. Cooperman describes. I agree that in all patients it is safe to insert a laparoscope, assess the status of the gallbladder, and initiate a trial dissection. We have set an arbitrary time limit of 60 minutes, at the end of which significant progress must have been made or the laparoscopic procedure is converted to an open cholecystectomy. The surgeon must not hesitate to convert the operation to a laparotomy should he feel uncomfortable with the progress of the procedure.

Laparoscopic surgery is limited by a lack of three-dimensional depth perception and the inability to perform manual palpation, thereby stripping the surgeon of some of his most important technical aids. Therefore dissection must be meticulous and the operative field must be viewed from both the dorsal and ventral aspects; manipulating the gallbladder superomedially and inferolaterally allows for optimal visualization. An important consideration in this group of patients in whom the anatomy may be partially obscured is the performance of intraoperative cholangiography to verify the status and anatomy of the biliary tree, which can compensate for the lack of direct visualization.

In selected cases of acutely inflamed gallbladders, additional instrument ports are necessary to provide the mandatory traction and countertraction; the surgeon should insert additional 5 mm laparoscopic sheaths if needed to apply upward traction on the gallbladder or downward traction on the transverse colon and duodenum. In the face of acute inflammation, the appropriate tissue planes are often easily dissected using what I term an "irrigating Kittner" technique. For this purpose I use the blunt tip of a spatulated cautery probe to manipulate the tissue while a continuous drip of heparinized saline containing cephalosporin (1 gm/L) is maintained through the lumen of the probe. The continuous irrigation clears the field of blood, bile, and other debris that may obscure vision. If the thick-walled gallbladder cannot be effectively grasped after decompression, we have found that with the use of 10 mm claw extracting forceps or a large three-pronged toothed grasper, traction can be maintained in most cases. When the cystic duct is inflamed, it is best not to rely solely on the placement of standard 9 mm clips but rather to suture the cystic duct with either a pre-tied slipknot or a suture looped around the duct and secured by manually tied knots.

At the conclusion of the operation, the operative field must be copiously irrigated until the fluid is clear; the irrigant is then aspirated. Placing the patient in a Trendelenburg position at the end of the operation allows the irrigant to return to the upper abdomen for aspiration. Drainage of the right upper quadrant is performed infrequently but can be done easily using a round 5 mm suction drain pulled through the operating port and exiting the lateral fundic port.

To summarize, in all patients with suspected acute cholecystitis, the gallbladder should be initially approached laparoscopically. Most patients can safely undergo laparoscopic cholecystectomy in this circumstance, but the surgeon must patiently and meticulously dissect the gallbladder from the portal structures to ensure that untoward complications do not occur. Intraoperative cholangiograms should be performed liberally if there is any doubt concerning the anatomy. The surgeon must not allow his ego to interfere with a rational evaluation of the surgical situation; in selected patients, circumstances will call for the procedure to be converted to an open cholecystectomy and the operation performed with binocular vision and manual palpation. When laparoscopic cholecystectomy for acute cholecystitis is successfully performed, patients may be discharged from the hospital within 24 to 48 hours and return to work within 7 to 10 days postoperatively.

Nathaniel J. Soper, M.D.

Assistant Professor of Surgery,
Washington University School of Medicine,
St. Louis, Mo.

• Invited Commentary •

Dr. Cooperman has provided an excellent review of the surgical approach to the "difficult" gallbladder encountered during laparoscopic cholecystectomy. He correctly points out that it is difficult to assess the severity of gallbladder inflammation preoperatively. For this reason it is our practice, as it is of Dr. Cooperman, to at least perform an initial diagnostic laparoscopy in patients presenting with acute cholecystitis. Once laparoscopic access is achieved, many of these difficult gallbladders can be successfully removed without risk or fear of injury to the extrahepatic biliary tree or major vascular structures.

Several important technical maneuvers can be performed that greatly assist in providing definitive treatment of acute cholecystitis under laparoscopic guidance. These maneuvers include decompression of the gallbladder, repositioning not only the laparoscope but also the graspers and dissectors to facilitate dissection, and placement of a large Jackson-Pratt drain into the subhepatic space.

Dr. Cooperman describes in detail a retrograde dissection of the acutely inflamed gallbladder, which begins at the fundus of the gallbladder and proceeds down toward the infundibulum, with eventual identification and exposure of the cystic duct, cystic artery, and common bile duct. It is stressed that all structures in the region of the porta hepatis and Calot's triangle should be clearly identified before ligation and transection.

At the University of Maryland we have also utilized retrograde dissection in several cases when the traditional approach to the cystic duct was obscured by severe inflammation. In deference to Dr. Cooperman's approach, we avoid if at all possible extensive dissection along the medial aspect of the gallbladder until the cystic duct has been clearly identified. We believe that dissection on the lateral aspect of the gallbladder is much safer and minimizes the risk of potential bile duct injury. A medial dissection, which is performed where the common hepatic duct and other vascular structures may be adherent to the wall of the gallbladder, may result in inadvertent injury to these structures.

In addition, although we use electrocautery for dissection of the gallbladder from the liver bed, we do not recommend the routine use of electrocautery during the identification of and dissection around the cystic duct, cystic artery, and common bile duct. We believe the potential for transmission of thermal energy and inadvertent injury to these structures is increased if electrocautery is used in this area.

Finally, one must keep in mind that the use of the retrograde approach brings the gallbladder and liver in much closer proximity to the colon and duodenum. The surgeon should be aware of this close approximation in order to avoid inadvertent injury with grasping forceps or the electrocautery or laser modalities.

Dr. Cooperman has provided excellent insight and "surgical secrets" for the removal of the acutely inflamed gallbladder using a laparoscopic approach. As is true with all surgical procedures, however, the safety and efficacy of any surgical procedure will be determined by the surgeon. As Dr. Cooperman has pointed out, all surgeons should have a low threshold for conversion of the procedure to an open cholecystectomy if it is impossible to accurately identify the appropriate anatomic structures.

Robert W. Bailey, M.D.

Assistant Professor, Department of Surgery,
University of Maryland School of Medicine,
Baltimore, Md.

·6·

Cholangiography
and Common Duct Stones

CHOLANGIOGRAPHY

Cholangiography has been an integral part of biliary surgery for more than 40 years. When no therapeutic alternatives were available for common duct stones other than open surgery, cholangiography was important in helping to determine if common duct stones were present or not. Whether common duct stones were overlooked at cholecystectomy or they re-formed de novo was immaterial because there was only one treatment option: surgical exploration of the common duct to remove the stone. If after an additional operation a stone still remained in the common duct, additional angst and surgery were distinct possibilities.

When percutaneous and endoscopic access to the common duct became possible, an overlooked or newly diagnosed common duct stone could now be observed, dissolved, pushed or pulled into the duodenum, or, if the stone was too large, fragmented by lithotripsy. The patient no longer was faced with surgery as the only choice. These noninvasive alternatives are as effective as surgery and more consumer friendly in that incisions and pain are avoided. As a result, some believe that routine cholangiography is no longer essential since the consequences of an overlooked stone are less ominous.

Selective cholangiography based on clinical criteria became popular as therapeutic options for common duct stones became more reliable. The indications for selective cholangiography have always been imprecise since common duct stones coexist with gallstones in at least 10% of cases.[1] Just as

113

the issue of the need for cholangiography with open cholecystectomy remains unresolved, so it has remained for cholangiography and laparoscopic cholecystectomy. Laparoscopic cholecystectomy is an ideal procedure for removing the gallbladder even if common duct stones are present. Other benefits offered by laparoscopic cholecystectomy, such as the chance to laparoscopically explore the common duct, are unanticipated bonuses. Thus three schools of thought have evolved regarding intraoperative cholangiography in laparoscopic surgery. First, there are those who advocate routine intraoperative cholangiography to portray common duct anatomy, limit anatomic surprises, determine if common duct stones are present, and attempt transcystic duct removal of stones with fluoroscopic or choledochoscopic guidance. If postoperative abdominal pain develops, the possibility of common duct stones has already been ruled out or verified with cholangiography. Second, there are those who favor selective cholangiography during laparoscopic surgery but believe that common duct stones are best left to endoscopists, who can remove them more precisely and deftly through the endoscope. They also believe routine identification of duct stones is unnecessary since many will pass spontaneously. Third, there are those who favor routine endoscopic studies before laparoscopic cholecystectomy. However, the low yield of common duct stones relative to the number of studies makes this economically impractical.[2-4]

For now laparoscopic removal of duct stones should be considered inconsistent and time consuming. Most surgeons prefer to have the common duct cleared of calculi before surgery. In this way the cholecystectomy is then definitive.

Indications

Many common duct stones pass without notice. No symptoms are manifested because the stones are smaller than the narrowest diameter of the common duct. The symptoms of common duct stone obstruction vary. If a stone significantly obstructs the common duct and pressure in the duct exceeds the pressure in the hepatic sinusoids, bacteria will back-diffuse into the sinusoids and cause cholangitis (manifested by chills, fever, and jaundice). There may be episodes of atypical biliary pain without objective signs. The presentation of jaundice, pruritus, dark urine, and abnormal liver function tests is more obvious. Severe abdominal pain and hyperamylasemia are strong indications that a stone has impacted or irritated the pancreatic duct during its passage. Dilated intrahepatic or extrahepatic ducts and a positive biliary scan are other signs that stones are present in the common bile duct.

Abnormal liver function tests, a recent history of jaundice, an elevated serum amylase level, or suggestive radiologic signs (e.g., dilated common duct) near the time laparoscopic surgery is scheduled warrant the performance of common duct studies. Whether these studies are done intraoperatively or preoperatively depends on the confidence and experience of the laparoscopic surgeon.

ENDOSCOPIC TREATMENT

The success rate for endoscopic retrieval of common duct stones as documented by cholangiography and postoperative course is greater than 90% and approaches 97% when lithotripsy is used for larger stones.[5-7] A recent study indicated a success rate with endoscopic retrograde cholangiopancreatography (ERCP) of only 35%.[8] This finding is in marked contrast to other recent studies that have demonstrated favorable results with endoscopic stone removal.[6,9-13] These studies have shown ERCP to have a decided advantage over open surgery in terms of lower morbidity, shorter hospital stay, and fewer residual common duct stones. Completion cholangiography must be performed after ERCP to document the status of the common duct.

There are few absolute contraindications to ERCP and a skilled endoscopist can overcome most relative contraindications. Relative contraindications include a previous Billroth II gastrectomy with a long afferent limb or a diverticulum near the ampulla. ERCP has also been less successful with a high stricture and intrahepatic duct stones. This situation is usually the result of a long-standing bile duct stricture, developing years after a cholecystectomy.

When common duct stones are suspected, an ERCP and stone extraction are scheduled prior to laparoscopic cholecystectomy (Fig. 6-1). Laparoscopic cholecystectomy is done the same day, presuming the endoscopic procedure is uneventful, without significant risk of bleeding or pancreatitis. If there are questionable findings or if acute pancreatitis arises, laparoscopy is delayed. Bowel gas introduced at ERCP has not been a problem during laparoscopy.

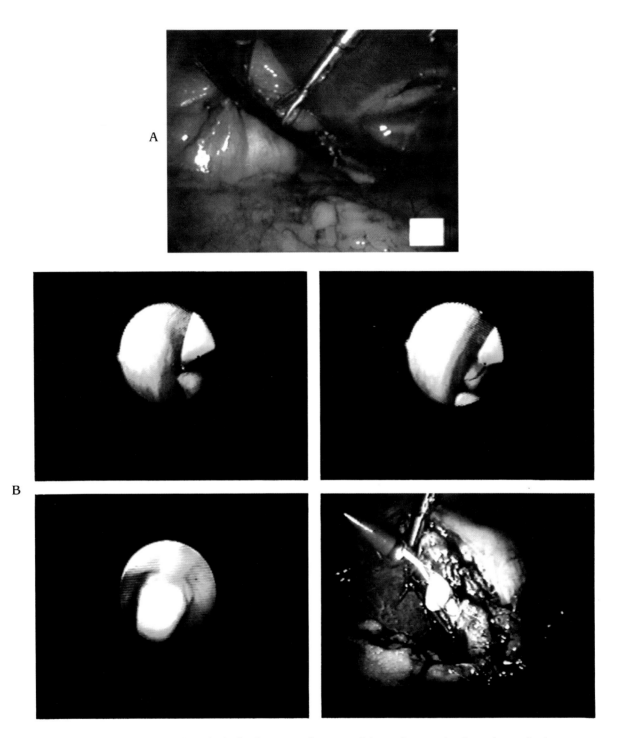

FIGURE 6-1 • **A,** The choledochoscope is passed into the cystic duct through the fundic port or the infundibular port. It is guided by the Olsen-cholangio clamp. **B,** Common duct stones are seen through the choledoscope and are removed with a basket. (Courtesy Douglas Olsen, M.D., Nashville, Tenn.)

If a common duct stone is identified but not retrieved at endoscopy, there are many treatment options. The endoscopist often does a "precut" on the sphincter and places a stent in the bile duct to prevent cholangitis and keep the sphincter open.[6,14] Endoscopy is then repeated 1 or 2 days later. The laparoscopic procedure is deferred until endoscopy is completed. An alternative is to perform open cholecystectomy and common duct exploration (my last choice). Other options include proceeding with laparoscopic cholecystectomy and leaving a transcystic duct catheter in the common duct. The stone can be removed postoperatively under fluoroscopy by an interventional radiologist. Another method is to open the common duct laparoscopically directly or to extend an incision in the cystic duct or the common duct and to use fluoroscopy or choledochoscopy to try to extract the stones laparoscopically with baskets. A T-tube can be placed in the common duct if the duct has been opened. The duct may be sutured if one is certain there are no residual stones. This requires direct suturing of the common duct and many surgeons may find the suturing time consuming and cumbersome.

Although impressive series of laparoscopic common duct exploration have been reported,[4] this must at present be balanced against the increase in operating time, the relative ease of endoscopic procedures, and the technical comfort for most surgeons. A more innovative approach involves contact lithotripsy, in which gallstones and common duct stones are fragmented, facilitating their passage and/or removal.

LAPAROSCOPIC CHOLANGIOGRAPHY

Several techniques of laparoscopic cholangiography are available, including cholecystocholangiogram, cystic duct cholangiogram, or direct puncture of the common duct (Fig. 6-2).

Cholecystocholangiogram

As long as the gallbladder is not tensely distended, the easiest type of cholangiogram to perform is a cholecystocholangiogram. An aspirating trocar is inserted through a 5 mm port and placed in the infundibulum of the gallbladder (Fig. 6-3). The gallbladder is injected with an undiluted contrast material; the bile will dilute the contrast material. The needle is then removed

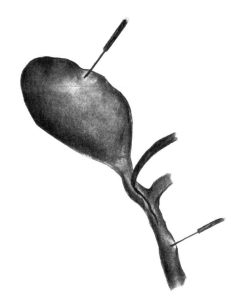

FIGURE 6-2 • Cholangiograms may be done through the gallbladder, cystic duct, or common duct.

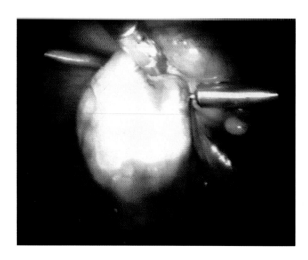

FIGURE 6-3 • A cholangiogram was taken by injecting undiluted contrast material directly into the gallbladder with a small trocar needle. The trocar was removed and then used to compress and empty the gallbladder. A fluorocholangiogram showed no stones in the common duct.

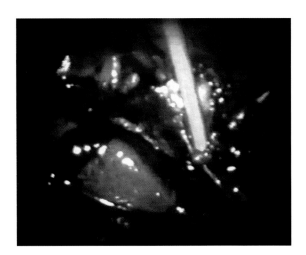

FIGURE 6-4 • A cholangiogram using a tapered catheter showed no stones in the bile duct. The beveled sheath fits directly into the cystic duct and a catheter is advanced into the lumen.

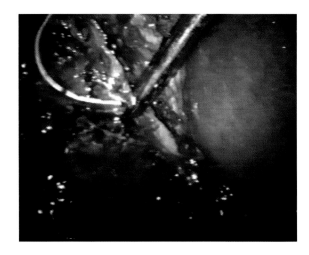

FIGURE 6-5 • A No. 5 feeding tube catheter was placed into the cystic duct and secured by an EndoLoop. A C-arm fluorocholangiogram was then obtained.

and the shaft of the trocar is used to compress and empty the gallbladder. This technique is simple and effective unless there is a stone obstructing the neck of the gallbladder and the cystic duct.

Cystic Duct Cholangiogram

Cholangiograms taken through the cystic duct have been the most popular method of cholangiography. Because the cystic duct is always dissected before the gallbladder is removed, the duct is easily exposed. With the magnification provided by the camera, cannulating the cystic duct during laparoscopy is not any more difficult than during the open technique.

In most cholecystectomies, the fundic port clamp can be used to maintain traction on the gallbladder, keeping the gallbladder elevated out of its fossa. Before the cystic duct is cannulated, it may be helpful to move the fundic port clamp to the lower part of the gallbladder where it can be used to provide upward traction on the gallbladder and the cystic duct. If the gallbladder is small, this clamp will provide satisfactory exposure of the cystic duct. The catheter, if made of soft plastic, may be difficult to thread into the cystic duct. New beveled cannulating catheters address this problem with a feature that allows them to self-secure into the cystic duct (Fig. 6-4). An inflatable balloon prevents bile leakage. The increased cost incurred with the use of these new catheters must be balanced against the shorter operating room time. These beveled catheters may also be introduced through the infundibular port into the cystic duct.

A plastic catheter, a central venous access catheter, or a ureteral catheter can also serve as a satisfactory conduit (Fig. 6-5). The only requirement is that the catheter be long enough to traverse the abdominal wall pneumoperitoneum and reach the cystic duct and the common duct. The catheter may be introduced through a needle placed in the abdominal wall. A clip is loosely applied to secure but not occlude the duct; saline solution is injected as the clip is applied to be certain that the duct lumen is not compromised. A new clamp is also available that secures the cystic duct and allows passage of a catheter through its lumen.

A C-arm fluorocholangiogram or an intraoperative cholangiogram is then obtained. The advantage of fluoroscopy is that it provides a continuous image on the screen. If the cholangiogram is negative, the surgeon can be more assured that stones are not present in the duct. If stones are present, an attempt is made to remove them under fluoroscopy by passing a Fogarty balloon catheter into the distal duct and inflating it (Fig. 6-6). A choledocho-scope may also be used if it will pass into the cystic duct. Further modifications of diagnostic catheters to allow baskets and balloons to pass through a channel into the common duct to extract calculi are anticipated.

If this technique cannot be done, the catheter is left in the duct and secured by an EndoLoop or tie passed around the cystic duct. The catheter and tract can then be used by a radiologist as a percutaneous pathway to remove the stone.

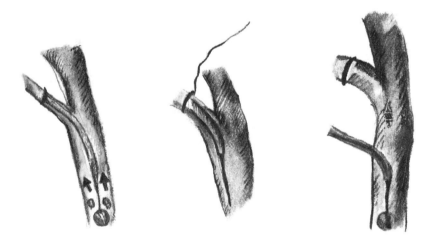

FIGURE 6-6 • If a common duct stone is found in the distal duct, several options are available. A balloon catheter may be passed into the distal duct guided by C-arm fluoroscopy, inflated, and the stones withdrawn. If the stones cannot be retrieved, a catheter may be left in the duct and secured by an EndoLoop or the common duct may be opened directly, stones removed, and the duct resutured.

Direct Common Duct Cholangiogram

Another method of obtaining a cholangiogram is through direct puncture of the common duct. The sheath of the operating port is removed and a scalp vein and attached tubing are inserted through the fascial opening into the common duct. The sheath is then replaced next to the tubing, and the tubing is connected to a syringe with contrast material. This method is used least frequently.

REFERENCES

1. Hermann RE, Vogt DP. Biliary system. In Davis JH, ed. Clinical Surgery. St. Louis: CV Mosby, 1987, pp 1637-1679.
2. Cotton PB. Endoscopic sphincterotomy before cholecystectomy. HPB Surg 1:244-247, 1989.
3. Reddick EJ, Olsen DO, Alexander W, et al. Laparoscopic laser cholecystectomy and choledocholithiasis. Surg Endosc 4:133-134, 1990.
4. Petelin J. Personal communication, Aug. 1991.
5. Siegel JH. Personal communication, Sept. 1991.
6. Siegel JH, Ben-Zvi JS, Pullano WF. Mechanical lithotripsy of common duct stones. Gastrointest Endosc 36(4):351-356, 1990.
7. Hansell DT, Millar MA, Murray WR, et al. Endoscopic sphincterotomy for bile duct stones in patients with intact gallbladders. Br J Surg 76(8):856-858, 1989.
8. Stain SC, Cohen H, Tsuishoysha M, et al. Choledocholithiasis: Endoscopic sphincterotomy or common bile duct exploration. Ann Surg 213:627-634, 1991.
9. Leese T, Neoptolemos JP, Baker AR, et al. Management of acute cholangitis and the impact of endoscopic sphincterotomy. Br J Surg 73:988-992, 1986.
10. Davidson BR, Neoptolemos JP, Carr-Locke DL. Endoscopic sphincterotomy for common bile duct calculi in patients with gallbladder in situ considered unfit for surgery. Gut 29:114-120, 1988.
11. Sivak MV Jr. Endoscopic management of bile duct stones. Am J Surg 158:228-240, 1989.
12. Zimmon DS. Alternatives to cholecystectomy and common duct exploration [editorial]. Am J Gastroenterol 83:1272-1273, 1988.
13. Cotton PB, Vallon AG. British experience with duodenoscopic sphincterotomy for removal of bile duct stones. Br J Surg 68:373-375, 1981.
14. Siegel JH, Ben-Zvi JS, Pullano WF. The needle knife: A valuable tool in diagnostic and therapeutic ERCP. Gastrointest Endosc 35:499-503, 1989.

• Invited Commentary •

When the laparoscopic management of common duct stones is discussed, the first issue that must be addressed is cholangiography. Even before laparoscopic cholecystectomy was introduced, the need for routine cholangiography was hotly debated. It is not surprising that even in the context of a laparoscopic approach, the controversy remains unresolved. Classic surgical teaching tells us that the anatomy must be clearly defined before any ductal structure, such as the cystic duct–common duct junction, is ligated or divided. During laparoscopic cholecystectomy, full visualization of this structure can sometimes be difficult, especially if there is acute or severe chronic inflammation. Excessive dissection in the portal triangle to delineate this anatomy can often lead to bleeding that is difficult to control and can possibly injure the duct. Using cholangiography, the surgeon has the ability to identify this anatomy without excessive dissection in Calot's triangle. The dissection can be carried out high on the neck of the gallbladder in an area that is safe and relatively avascular. Not only is the anatomy then clearly identified, but the presence of any stones in either the cystic duct stump or the common duct can be evaluated. Intraoperative management of common duct stones is possible only if they are identified at the time of the surgery. But even postoperative management using ERCP is facilitated with a good intraoperative cholangiogram.

Another key issue is the avoidance of unnecessary common duct exploration—not via open choledochotomy, but via ERCP. ERCP is a costly and time-consuming procedure that should not be performed without the proper indication. The performance of intraoperative cholangiograms certainly reduces the need for both preoperative and postoperative ERCPs.

The actual management of common duct stones varies according to when the stones are detected: preoperatively or intraoperatively. Approximately 15% of patients who present with gallbladder disease have common duct stones.[1] Approximately one third of these patients have no preoperative indications of choledocholithiasis.[1] Patients who are identified preoperatively as being at high risk for common duct stones should undergo preoperative ERCP for both diagnosis and management. If the stones cannot be removed in this fashion or if complications develop, the surgeon then has the option of proceeding with a more classic approach.

When the stones are found intraoperatively, I opt to attempt to remove them through the cystic duct stump using choledochoscopy. I do not favor laparoscopic choledochotomy because it violates one of the principles of minimally invasive surgery—rapid postoperative return to normal activities. When choledochotomy is performed, a T-tube is inserted and should not be removed for at least 10 to 14 days. In contrast, not only can postoperative ERCP treat the same stone, but the patient is able to return to work as quickly as a patient who has undergone a simple laparoscopic cholecystectomy, and a tube draining the common duct is not necessary.

When an attempt is made to remove stones through the cystic duct, it must be kept in mind that postoperative ERCP offers a good alternative. Excessive time or risk should not be taken to attempt to remove stones at laparoscopic cholecystectomy. If the stones cannot be easily managed through the cystic duct, then the laparoscopic cholecystectomy should be completed and postoperative ERCP performed to clear stones from the duct. Only if there is a contraindication to postoperative ERCP would I consider laparoscopic choledochotomy. Approaching treatment with this philosophy, I have not had any patient require reoperation for removal of retained stones, and I have been successful in managing common duct stones with a minimally invasive technique in more than 92% of my patients.

Douglas O. Olsen, M.D., F.A.C.S.

Assistant Clinical Professor of Surgery,
Vanderbilt University,
Nashville, Tenn.

REFERENCE

1. Sabiston DC Jr. Textbook of Surgery: The Biological Basis of Modern Surgical Practice, 13th ed. Philadelphia: WB Saunders, 1986.

• Invited Commentary •

Ductal evaluation during cholecystectomy has been a topic of discussion and sometimes controversy for over 100 years. Indeed, the first open cholecystectomy was performed in 1882 by Langenbuch, the first successful common duct stone removal completed by Courvoiser in 1890, and intraoperative cholangiography introduced by Mirizzi in 1932. Innumerable parleys exploring the pros and cons of a variety of approaches to the problem have been convened.

Dr. Cooperman clearly summarizes the prevailing views on laparoscopic cholecystectomy. I would like to address specific issues in each school of thought regarding cholangiography. First, let us consider the use of routine preoperative endoscopic retrograde cholangiopancreatography (ERCP). As Dr. Cooperman has indicated, this approach would prove incredibly costly if applied uniformly to all laparoscopic cholecystectomy patients. In addition, the potential for complications resulting from ERCP (e.g., pancreatitis) would seem to preclude the routine performance of such a low-yield procedure (i.e., 10% incidence of common duct stones). Second, those who believe that common duct stones are best left alone by surgeons and that routine cholangiography is therefore unnecessary are possibly overlooking the fact that during the early development of ERCP, a rather high failure rate for common duct stone extraction occurred. Admittedly, endoscopists are today much more adept in their manipulations of the distal duct than they were in the early days. The point, however, is that general surgeons will not become adept at cholangiography and common duct exploration if they do not attempt it! Having performed over 640 cholangiograms and over 50 laparoscopic common duct explorations in over 750 laparoscopic cholecystectomies, I can assure you that (1) it becomes easier with each case; (2) cholangiography usually adds approximately 15 minutes and laparoscopic common duct exploration usually adds less than 30 minutes of actual operating time once the equipment is ready; (3) patients benefit from leaving the hospital in less than 24 hours, cured of their biliary tract disease without the need for an expensive return trip for ERCP; and (4) patients are relieved of the lifelong risk of possible complications from a sphincterotomy. Third, there are those who recommend routine intraoperative cholangiography. As Dr. Cooperman has pointed out, such a practice defines the anatomy so that surgical misadventure is improbable and evaluates the ductal system for stones or other pathologic conditions. The other most obvious reason for suggesting routine use of laparoscopic cholangiography early in a surgeon's laparoscopic experience is to establish proficiency in the maneuver itself. Thereafter, if a surgeon suspects that there is a very low chance of common duct pathologic conditions (i.e., large stones and small ducts), then a more selective approach to intraoperative cholangiography may be appropriate. There is one situation, however, in which I believe intraoperative cholangiography is imperative: in the patient who has undergone preoperative ERCP and stone extraction. I have personally found and removed common duct stones laparoscopically in a patient who had undergone a previous successful ERCP stone extraction and who had normal cholangiograms following the procedure.

The method of cholangiography varies from surgeon to surgeon. Two basic approaches have evolved: the portal technique developed by Olsen and Reddick in 1989 and the percutaneous technique developed by Petelin in 1990. Modifications of both approaches have been used to gain access to the peritoneal cavity and the ductal system. Obviously, I prefer the percutaneous technique. Quite simply it involves the placement of a 14-gauge polyethylene catheter 2 inches in length through the abdominal wall. It is located 2.5 cm medial to the midclavicular port and is inserted in a slightly cephalad direction. Through this fifth port, any plastic catheter may be inserted and manipulated into the cystic duct with forceps inserted through the medial epigastric port. The catheter is fixed into position in the duct with a clip. Once the catheter is removed from the duct, it is withdrawn from the peritoneal cavity and the sheath is capped with a heparin-lock style cap, which prevents the loss of carbon dioxide from the abdomen and avoids the accumulation of gas in the subcutaneous tissues that might occur if the catheter were completely removed. Additionally, the sheath may subsequently be used for placement of a 4 Fr Fogarty catheter into the ductal system for dilation and/ or removal of debris.

Common duct stones may be treated by any of the methods discussed by Dr. Cooperman. Each approach has merits and limitations. I believe that as a surgeon becomes more expert in his laparoscopic skills, his approach to the common duct will change. For example, early in one's experience, if common duct stones are strongly suspected, then preoperative ERCP and stone extraction is usually preferred. If stones are discovered during laparoscopic cholangiography, then either open common duct exploration or postoperative ERCP is selected. As one gains confidence, however, even those patients suspected of having common duct stones preoperatively may be taken directly to the operating room for laparoscopic cholecystectomy and laparoscopic common duct exploration, with the expectation of successful clearance of the biliary system in over 93% of cases (based on my personal experience). This approach avoids the expense and morbidity of preoperative ERCP. It is important for the surgeon to clearly understand his own approach to these problems and to explain to the patient the possible scenarios that might be enacted if common duct stones are detected.

It behooves all biliary tract surgeons to become as adept at treating biliary ductal problems laparoscopically as they are at treating them in open surgery. We do not need to relinquish our ability to treat the common duct to other minimally invasive practitioners.

Joseph B. Petelin, M.D., F.A.C.S.

Clinical Assistant Professor of Surgery,
Department of Surgery, University of
Kansas School of Medicine,
Kansas City, Kan.

·7·

Pancreatitis

With cholecystitis, until the laparoscope is introduced into the patient's abdomen, the degree of operative difficulty is unknown. In contrast, the difficulties with gallstone pancreatitis are recognized preoperatively. Its management has stirred some controversy since its course may be unpredictable. This chapter describes my present approach to gallstone pancreatitis and discusses options and alternatives.

PRESENTING SYMPTOMS

Ninety percent of patients with gallstone pancreatitis have gallstone hyperamylasemia, which is a transient rise in the amylase level as the stone, coursing down the bile duct, irritates the pancreatic duct. This elevation in amylase level is benign, self-limiting, and of little consequence. In these patients with gallstone hyperamylasemia, abdominal pain, if present, rapidly subsides. Their appetite returns and they feel well within hours to days. Most important, the pancreas incurs no damage. However, in 10% of patients with pancreatitis, the disease is protracted and severe, marked by renal, respiratory, or septic complications.[1] This disease carries a far different and more serious outcome, and consideration of laparoscopic cholecystectomy is deferred until the patient has recovered. Rarely, the presentation may be asymptomatic hyperamylasemia found on routine blood tests in patients with known gallbladder calculi. In these patients, the common bile duct is small, and the stones that pass from the gallbladder are of sufficient size to irritate the pancreatic duct as they pass through the distal bile duct but small enough to pass unimpeded into the intestine. This presentation is not considered clinical pancreatitis.

TREATMENT

In patients with gallstone hyperamylasemia, when the hyperamylasemia and abdominal pain resolve, preoperative endoscopic retrograde cholangio-pancreatography (ERCP) and endoscopic retrieval of stones (if necessary) are performed (Fig. 7-1). In skilled hands, the procedure is both diagnostic and therapeutic and involves less pain and morbidity than open surgery. Its success rate for clearing duct stones is greater than 90%.[2] In most cases a duct stone will not be found because it has passed into the intestine.

Patients with severe pancreatitis who require large volumes of fluid and ventilatory or renal support often have a protracted course. In these patients, the amylase level ranges from normal to elevated. A stone lodged in the bile duct is most easily managed by ERCP and endoscopic removal. With this type of life-threatening pancreatitis, open surgery, with its associated high mortality and morbidity, should be avoided. However, surgery may be required for septic complications.

Timing of Treatment

Only recently have questions centered on the timing of endoscopy and biliary surgery for pancreatitis. Before the introduction of endoscopic studies, there was no choice but to proceed with cholecystectomy and then intraoperatively either explore the common duct routinely or perform a cholangiogram. Based on the findings, a decision regarding further duct exploration was then made. However, the availability of endoscopic studies has altered the approach to biliary surgery today.

It was once thought by some that open surgery early in the course of pancreatitis might prevent disease progression.[3] However, ERCP and endo-scopic retrieval of stones is now recognized as a safe and sensible alternative approach.[2,4-7] It simplifies for the laparoscopic surgeon the intraoperative decision of whether or not to explore the common duct. The longer one waits

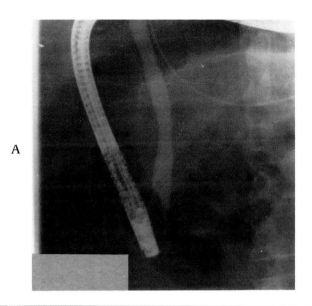

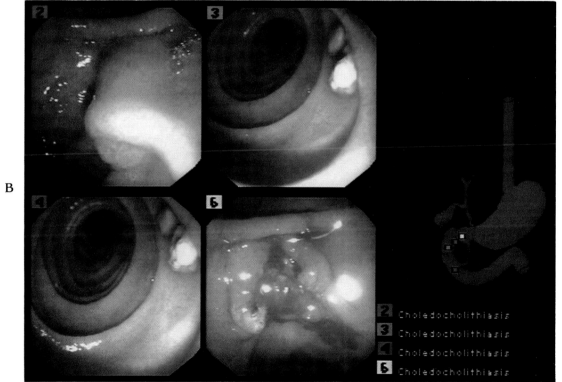

FIGURE 7-1 • **A,** An ERCP film showing stones in the distal bile duct. A bulging papilla with a stone behind it was the cause of gallstone pancreatitis. **B,** After a sphincterotomy was performed, stones were removed by basketing. (Courtesy Jerome Siegel, M.D., New York, N.Y.)

to examine the common bile duct after gallstone pancreatitis presents, the lower the incidence of duct stones since time is allowed for their spontaneous passage. Forty-eight to 72 hours after the onset of gallstone hyperamylasemia, the incidence of common duct stones is 63% to 78%.[7] Yet 1 week to 1 month later, the incidence falls to 3% to 33%.[7] The high success rate and low complication rate with ERCP and endoscopic sphincterotomy make it the treatment of choice for common duct stones in gallstone pancreatitis. Randomization of patients with mild and severe pancreatitis has shown that early endoscopic intervention is safe and may in fact be associated with fewer sequelae than open surgery.[7] Obviously, the assistance of an experienced, confident endoscopist is essential.

Routine vs. Selective Biliary Endoscopy

Some hold that the logical extension of biliary endoscopy is its routine preoperative use for all cholecystectomy patients. This practice may be valid in centers where intraoperative studies are inaccurate or difficult to obtain. It reduces the number of unnecessary common duct explorations, reduces the risk of missing stones intraoperatively, and eliminates a sometimes frequent source of intraoperative frustration—having to perform intraoperative cholangiography. These advantages must be balanced against cost, a small but definite incidence of pancreatitis resulting from the performance of endoscopy, and a greater than 90% negative yield.[7] I have become more selective about ERCP and its application in laparoscopic surgery: I obtain ERCPs before laparoscopic cholecystectomy only in patients with recent episodes of gallstone pancreatitis or in those suspected of having duct stones.

An additional option in a patient with a normal-sized common duct who has a history of pancreatitis is to obtain an intraoperative laparoscopic cholangiogram. Intraoperative cholangiography avoids the expense of an ERCP and is as effective in detecting stones. If stones are present in the common bile duct, they often can be retrieved through the cystic duct with either a balloon catheter or choledochoscope (see Chapter 6). If this method of retrieval is unsuccessful, a catheter may be left in the common duct through the cystic duct to provide access for the interventional radiologist or endoscopist.

CLINICAL EXPERIENCE

In a 10-month period in 1990, 10 of 220 consecutive patients who underwent laparoscopic cholecystectomy had a history of pancreatitis (5%).[6] Presentations were varied and wide ranging. In two of the 10 with known gallstones, hyperamylasemia was detected with routine blood tests during health examinations. They were otherwise asymptomatic and did not have biliary colic or abdominal pain. Six patients were previously hospitalized from 48 to 96 hours for acute abdominal pain secondary to acute pancreatitis from cholecystitis. In all six patients, the enzyme abnormalities corrected spontaneously and they were dismissed from the hospital. Two patients suffered acute episodes of biliary colic and pancreatitis, and open surgery was recommended. In both, elevated pancreatic enzymes corrected spontaneously. An additional patient had severe pancreatitis with pseudocysts and respiratory insufficiency. He underwent a diagnostic study with percutaneous drainage of the bile duct. He has required several months of hospitalization to recover from the respiratory and septic complications of pancreatitis, which have been managed nonoperatively.

The bile duct was studied in all 10 patients: eight by ERCP (two patients had stones, which were removed by ERCP) and two by intraoperative cholangiography (negative in both).

These 10 patients in our series fared no differently than the 210 patients without pancreatitis who had laparoscopic cholecystectomy. Two patients were treated on an ambulatory basis, seven remained hospitalized for 24 hours or less, and one patient remained hospitalized for 3 days because of her advanced age (74 years) and a history of stroke.

•   •   •

Gallstone pancreatitis should not be a contraindication to laparoscopic cholecystectomy. Problems with common duct stones can be dealt with preoperatively by ERCP and intraoperatively with cholangiography.

REFERENCES

1. Cooperman AM, Hoerr SO, Reed R. Surgery of the Pancreas—A Text and Atlas. St. Louis: CV Mosby, 1978, pp 89-95.
2. Chen FC, Hill DA, Hugh TB, et al. Endoscopic management of gallstone pancreatitis. Aust N Z J Surg 61(2):161-162, 1991.
3. Skinner DB. Should early surgical intervention be routinely recommended in the management of gallstone pancreatitis? In Gitnick G, ed. Controversies in Gastroenterology. London: Churchill Livingstone, 1984, pp 197-203.
4. Safrany L, Cotton PB. A preliminary report: Urgent duodenoscopic sphincterotomy for acute gallstone pancreatitis. Surgery 89:424-428, 1981.
5. Van Spuy DS. Endoscopic sphincterotomy in the management of gallstone pancreatitis. Endoscopy 13:25-26, 1986.
6. Cooperman AM, Siegel J, Neff R, et al. Gallstone pancreatitis—Combined endoscopic and laparoscopic approaches. J Laparoendosc Surg 1:115-117, 1991.
7. Neoptolemus JP, London NJ, James D, et al. Controlled trial of urgent endoscopic retrograde cholangiopancreatography and endoscopic sphincterotomy versus conservative treatment for acute pancreatitis due to gallstones. Lancet 2:979-983, 1988.

·8·

Carcinoma

An unfortunate but uncommon finding during laparoscopic cholecystectomy is unsuspected carcinoma of the gallbladder. Can it be adequately treated at the laparoscopic procedure? What should be done?

Consideration of the use of laparoscopic surgery for the treatment of gall-bladder cancer should be tempered by knowledge of the limited survival rate associated with this cancer and the natural history of the disease. The overall 5-year survival rate following surgery for gallbladder cancer is only 5%.[1] When unsuspected gallbladder cancer is discovered at the time of cholecys-tectomy, it is usually detected by the pathologist when the routine micro-scopic sections are examined postoperatively. When tumors are grossly evident at surgery, they are usually in the late stage and cure is unlikely.

When the carcinoma is discovered by chance, laparoscopic cholecystec-tomy, like open cholecystectomy, has been found to be therapeutic if the tumor is confined to the superficial layers of the gallbladder wall. Treatment for the incidentally discovered gallbladder cancer that is deeply invasive is controversial. The question as to whether radical reoperative surgery is curative or increases survival rates is unsettled.[2,3] Those who advocate re-section of the liver margin and lymph nodes believe survival data justify this approach. The extent of nodal dissection undertaken ranges from only regional nodes (hilum and common duct) to hilar, paraductal, and para-aortic nodes. Others think the biologic behavior of gallbladder cancer and the limited survival rate are not affected by additional surgery, and therefore further treatment is futile.

Chemotherapy and radiation therapy have achieved only sporadic success, thus they do not offer a significant hope for cure at present.

LITERATURE REVIEW

It is difficult to draw conclusions from a literature analysis since most reports involve small numbers of patients, are weighted heavily toward advanced tumors, lack randomization, and are biased toward surgical treatment. Cases in which gallbladder cancer has been incidentally found are few. If patients have done well after reoperative "extended" surgery (i.e., resection of lymph nodes and liver), is it because of the treatment or the behavior of the tumor?

A report from England of 29 patients with gallbladder cancer indicated that in only two of 21 operated patients were the cancers found incidentally during cholecystectomy.[4] Although it was possible to resect the tumor in 14 patients, only one patient survived 5 years. The mean postoperative survival time was only 6.6 months, which reflects the late stage at which the disease was detected.

In a Chilean study, 15 of 52 invasive gallbladder cancers detected in a 2-year period did not extend to the serosal layer.[5] Four of the 15 patients whose tumors were confined to the mucosa did not undergo additional surgery, whereas the remaining 11 patients underwent lymph node dissection (the tumors did not extend through the gallbladder) and wedge resection of liver in the porta hepatis. In seven of the 11 patients, the primary tumor was found only on microscopic sectioning of the gallbladder. Five of the 11 patients who underwent lymph node dissection had nodal involvement and three of these five also had liver involvement. Long-term results were not reported. This study will be of greater value when follow-up is extended for a longer period, but it does indicate that occult or small tumors can metastasize to lymph nodes and the liver.

A 13-year review from the Mayo Clinic of 111 patients with gallbladder cancer indicated that nearly 60% of the patients had late-stage tumors at the time of presentation.[2] The median survival rate was 0.5 year and the 5-year survival rate was 13%. Although tumor stage and tumor grade were predictive of outcome, DNA and tumor ploidy were not. Of interest is a subset of patients (36%) whose treatment was open simple cholecystectomy (20%) or radical cholecystectomy (nodal dissection plus surrounding liver [16%]). Cure was considered possible in all of these patients. Median survival time was 3.6 years after radical surgery and 0.8 year after cholecystectomy, but the 5-year survival rates were comparable (33% vs. 32%). The conclusion that radical cholecystectomy may benefit individual patients but does not offer a long-term survival advantage is sobering.

Reports from Japan favor a more aggressive approach, occasionally involving a combined pancreaticoduodenal resection; liver resection; and portal vein, bile duct, and nodal resections.[6,7] Occasional long-term survivors and a consistently low morbidity and mortality are the supporting evidence for this approach.

An analysis of prognostic factors in 36 gallbladder cancer patients after "curative" resection indicated survival varied inversely with depth of tumor penetration.[8] The worst survival rates were associated with tumors that extended to the serosa of the gallbladder. All tumors limited to the mucosa and nearly all confined to the muscularis were papillary rather than nodular. Nodular tumors were more infiltrative than papillary tumors and had a worse prognosis. The deeper the tumor penetration, the greater the venous, lymphatic, and perineural invasion. For patients with tumors that did not penetrate the subserosa, a longer survival time was noted after extended surgery than after cholecystectomy alone. Aggressive surgery favored survival.

ILLUSTRATIVE CASES

I have encountered two cases of gallbladder cancer in 300 laparoscopic cholecystectomies. Both presentations were unanticipated and represent both ends of the spectrum in terms of malignancy.

Case 1

A 54-year-old woman presented with the recent onset of acute upper abdominal pain and a right upper quadrant mass. An ultrasound detected gallstones and an enlarged gallbladder. The white blood cell count was elevated. Hydrops was suspected. During laparoscopic cholecystectomy, a large cancer involving the gallbladder, right lobe of the liver, and transverse colon was found. Biopsies were performed and the laparoscopic procedure terminated. The tumor was considered unresectable and the patient was referred for oncologic evaluation. Angiography confirmed the presence of an extensive unresectable tumor. The patient underwent systemic chemo-therapy, but she did poorly as the disease progressed inexorably.

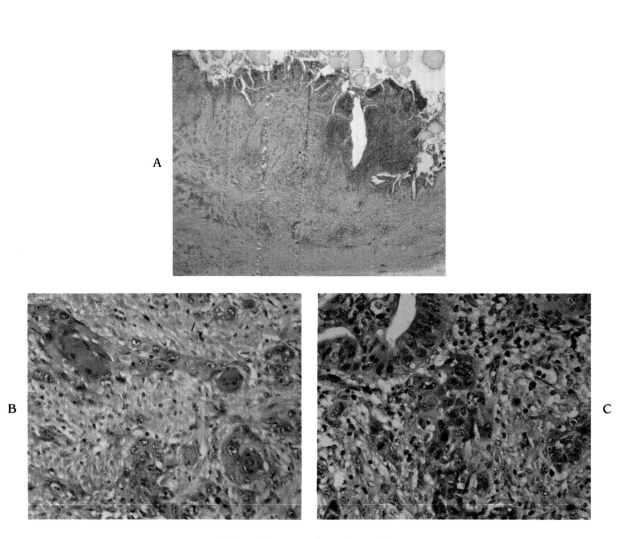

FIGURE 8-1 • **A,** An unanticipated <1 cm invasive adenosquamous cancer in the infundibulum was discovered on routine sectioning of the gallbladder (hematoxylin-eosin, x10). **B** and **C,** The cancer had invaded to the serosa but not through the wall. Squamous and glandular components were detected (hematoxylin-eosin, x40).

Case 2

A 32-year-old woman 6 months postpartum underwent laparoscopic chole-cystectomy for recurrent acute cholecystitis. At laparoscopic cholecystec-tomy, an impacted infundibular stone was found in the neck of the gallblad-der. The cholecystectomy specimen included a cuff of peritoneum between the gallbladder and liver. During routine sectioning of the gallbladder a <1 cm adenosquamous carcinoma at the infundibulum was found. The tumor penetrated through the muscularis mucosa to the serosa but not through it (Fig. 8-1). The cystic duct was not involved. A cystic duct node was examined and found to be negative for tumor.

Particularly disturbing in this case is the patient's young age and the risk of metastasis. Since the tumor was small and in the infundibulum, which was separated from the liver bed by a gross margin, nodal metastases along the common duct are a concern. The lack of a reliable systemic agent limits the value of a staging procedure if the lymph nodes are positive. The limited survival rate at 5 years (32% to 35%) even after curative procedures echoes this conclusion.[3] Equally frustrating is the controversial and unproven role of additional therapy. Perhaps laparoscopic nodal resection would be fruitful and would avoid a laparotomy in this situation.

Little has been written about adenosquamous carcinoma, a variant of adenocarcinoma. Although the presence of the squamous component raises the possibility that chronic inflammation is a premalignant condition, the patient's young age and short history of cholecystitis do not support this theory in this case.

CONCLUSION

The recent literature does much to subclassify and analyze gallbladder cancer, but it does little to resolve the issues concerning the extent of resection and the effectiveness of adjuvant therapy. Until these issues are resolved, the triumph of hope over reality will continue to be presented in the literature. Early diagnosis and aggressive therapy, which have been the unfulfilled keys to cancer treatment for decades, are not enough for gallblad-der cancer. Decision making in individual cases remains imprecise and frustrating for a disease with a limited prognosis.

Most cases of gallbladder cancer are discovered at surgery. Most "early" or occult gallbladder cancers are discovered days after open cholecystectomy is performed and the unsuspected finding is a shock to the patient, surgeon, and pathologist. Although laparoscopic cholecystectomy avoids an incision to establish the unsuspected diagnosis, it is no more and no less curative than open cholecystectomy. The temptation is to reexplore the operative area with the laparoscope and excise paraductal nodes. I think (allowing time for instrumentation to be developed) thorough laparoscopic exploration of the portal and ductal areas will be possible in the future to stage the lesion and perhaps effect statistical benefit regarding survival. When effective systemic therapy becomes available, a rationale will exist to support this approach.

REFERENCES

1. Adson MA. Carcinoma of the gallbladder. Surg Clin North Am 53:1203-1216, 1975.
2. Donohue JH, Nagorney DM, Grant CS, et al. Carcinoma of the gallbladder. Does radical resection improve outcome? Arch Surg 125(2):237-241, 1990.
3. Nakamura S, Sakaguchi S, Suzuki S, et al. Aggressive surgery for carcinoma of the gallbladder. Surgery 106(3):467-473, 1989.
4. Burgess P, Murphy PD, Clague MB. Adenocarcinoma of the gallbladder: A 5-year review of outcome in Newcastle Upon Tyne. J R Soc Med 84:54-61, 1991.
5. de Aretxabala X, Roa I, Araya JC, et al. Operative findings in patients with early forms of gallbladder cancer. Br J Surg 77(3):291-293, 1990.
6. Kumada K, Ozawa K, Shimahara Y, et al. Truncoumbilical bypass of the portal vein in radical resection of biliary tract tumor involving the hepatic duct confluence. Br J Surg 77(7):749-751, 1990.
7. Tsunoda T, Tsuchiya R, Harada N, et al. The surgical treatment for carcinoma of the gallbladder—Rationale of the second-look operation for inapparent carcinoma. Jpn J Surg 6(17):478-486, 1987.
8. Ouchi K, Owada Y, Matsuno S, et al. Prognostic factors in the surgical treatment of gallbladder carcinoma. Surgery 101:731, 1987.

• Invited Commentary •

The question as to how best to approach carcinoma of the gallbladder when encountered during laparoscopic cholecystectomy is raised by the case presentations in this chapter. If unequivocal efficacy for a specific procedure were established by a randomized clinical trial, the role of laparoscopic surgery would be clear: duplicate the treatment of choice laparoscopically. However, optimal operative management for carcinoma of the gallbladder remains undefined. Without a widely accepted and proven therapy, a rational surgical approach is to adapt treatment to the extent or stage of disease. Three basic clinical scenarios of carcinoma of the gallbladder might be encountered laparoscopically: (1) advanced disease, (2) occult disease, or (3) obvious disease without apparent metastases. What are the reasonable treatment options for each scenario based on current treatment results in the literature?

First, unsuspected advanced disease is rarely encountered. If performed by an experienced radiologist, modern preoperative imaging for calculous biliary tract disease, particularly with ultrasonography, will almost always reveal a gallbladder mass or focal-wall thickening with liver metastases or obvious regional lymphadenopathy. False-negative imaging can occur from small peritoneal implants or hepatic metastases. When advanced disease is recognized at laparoscopy, histologic confirmation through biopsy is essential. In general, laparoscopic cholecystectomy should only be performed if the gallbladder is unequivocally symptomatic and the local and regional extent of the cancer is not technically prohibitive. In fact, effective palliation is rarely possible in patients with advanced disease.

Second, the scenario of clinically occult disease, whether pathologically confirmed intraoperatively by frozen section or postoperatively confirmed by permanent section, poses a more difficult clinical dilemma. However, a rational approach can be developed on the basis of disease stage or more specifically by the T classification of the TNM definition of carcinoma of the gallbladder.[1] As noted by Dr. Cooperman, advanced disease is typically associated with transmural extension of the cancer. Current data show that survival of patients whose tumors lack transmural extension is significantly greater than that of patients whose tumors demonstrate such extension. Indeed, depth of tumor invasion (T) is a key prognostic factor for patients with carcinoma of the gallbladder. Survival decreases further as the tumor grossly invades adjacent viscera and structures (T3 and T4 disease).[2,3] What then is the treatment algorithm based on depth of invasion? If careful histologic examination fails to identify transmural involvement, laparoscopic cholecystectomy alone is appropriate. Sampling of the cystic duct and pericholedochal lymph nodes is appropriate for further staging if the tumor is recognized on frozen section intraoperatively. If pathologic confirmation is delayed, no further intervention is required. Conversion of a laparoscopic cholecystectomy to an open abdominal procedure for regional lymphadenectomy and possible liver resection is indicated for transmural involvement (T3 or T4 disease) or regional lymph node involvement (N1a) confirmed by sampling. Laparoscopic cholecystectomy alone, with or without lymph node sampling, is appropriate for Tis, T1, or T2 disease.

Third, the operating surgeon may encounter an obvious carcinoma of the gallbladder based on gross laparoscopic characteristics. Clearly, laparoscopic abdominal examination is indicated. If that examination fails to reveal distant disease, open cholecystectomy anticipating regional lymphadenectomy and hepatic resection if necessary should be advised on the basis of current survival data.[2,3]

In conclusion, the local and regional extent of carcinoma of the gallbladder is the primary determinant of the surgical approach. If disease is occult and transmural involvement is absent, laparoscopic cholecystectomy is sufficient treatment. However, if transmural extension exists without distant disease, conversion to an open procedure, which addresses the local and regional extent of the disease, is indicated. As laparoscopic techniques advance, perhaps laparoscopic approaches will be equivalent to open procedures. Until such developments occur, disease stage dictates the technical approach.

David M. Nagorney, M.D.
*Associate Professor of Surgery,
Mayo Medical School, Mayo Clinic,
Rochester, Minn.*

REFERENCES

1. American Joint Committee on Cancer. Gallbladder. In Beahrs OH, Henson DE, Hutter RVP, et al., eds. Manual for Staging of Cancer, 3rd ed. Philadelphia: JB Lippincott, 1988, pp 93-95.
2. Gagner M, Rossi RL. Radical operations for carcinoma of the gallbladder: Present status in North America. World J Surg 15:344-347, 1991.
3. Donohue JH, Nagorney DM, Grant CS, et al. Carcinoma of the gallbladder: Does radical resection improve outcome? Arch Surg 125:237-241, 1990.

·III·

Complications and Outcome

·9·

Complications: Creative Solutions

Preview

- Prevention is the best method of dealing with complications.
- Insertion of trocars and ports, which is a blind procedure, requires adequate pneumoperitoneum and a light touch.
- Bleeding can be controlled without converting the operation to an open cholecystectomy.
- Spilled stones can be retrieved and removed laparoscopically.

The surge of popularity enjoyed by laparoscopic cholecystectomy has been tempered by a learning curve that has been associated with a higher morbidity than that for open cholecystectomy. Complications may occur when obtaining laparoscopic access, during insufflation, or during the cholecystectomy itself.

Although laparoscopic procedures can be converted to open cholecystectomy, this happens more often after an intraoperative complication develops rather than as an anticipatory step. Thus when difficulties are encountered, the fallback option of open cholecystectomy should unhesitatingly be exercised.

GENERAL RISK FACTORS

Laparoscopy is associated with less risk than laparotomy. However, laparoscopy is not without risk, particularly in compromised patients with cardiac, pulmonary, or renal disease. Patients at high risk from local factors include those with ascites (the bowel may rise with the ascitic fluid and compromise pneumoperitoneum); previous abdominal surgery; gastric, bowel, or bladder distention; and uncorrected bleeding disorders.

CARDIAC COMPLICATIONS

The most frequent cardiac complication is arrhythmia. Other cardiac complications are fortunately rare. The incidence of arrhythmia when carbon dioxide is used as the insufflating agent is as high as 20%.[1-4] Arrhythmias are transient and generally do not affect the operative procedure. Hypoventilation, another possible cause of cardiac complications, is not common with laparoscopy, particularly when general anesthesia is used.

PULMONARY COMPLICATIONS

Pulmonary complications include aspiration, embolism, pneumothorax, and subcutaneous emphysema. Aspiration secondary to reflux is not common. Recent studies have shown no increase in esophageal reflux with the increased intra-abdominal pressure caused by pneumoperitoneum.[5] Postoperative pulmonary changes are less frequent after laparoscopic cholecystectomy than after open laparotomy and tend to be less significant.

TROCAR AND NEEDLE INJURIES

Not surprisingly, significant complications can be caused by the blind introduction of needles and trocars into the abdomen. When an untoward force is applied to a needle or trocar, a forceful pushing motion occurs upon entry into the abdomen. The sharp tip of these instruments can puncture retroperitoneal vessels, stomach, small bowel, colon, and bladder. The retroperitoneal vessels are injured less often than the other structures because they are covered by viscera, which act as a protective sheath and are injured first. Significant and sometimes fatal injuries have occurred when a trocar pierced major vascular structures, particularly the aorta, vena cava, or iliac vessels. These injuries are infrequent but not unknown during a laparoscopic career.[6-12] In a recent study, 25% of laparoscopists noted that at least one of their patients had experienced a needle or trocar injury during laparoscopy.[13] A survey of German hospitals and clinics indicated a morbidity of 1.97% in nearly 250,000 gynecologic laparoscopic procedures caused by injury with nondisposable needles and trocars.[6] The most frequent injury was a Veress needle or a trocar injury to a viscus or major blood vessel.

Treatment

Trocar injuries require immediate repair. If the trocar has injured the bladder or an isolated single loop of small bowel, either the repair can be performed laparoscopically or the small bowel can be pulled onto the abdominal wall, repaired, and replaced in the abdomen before continuing the procedure.[14] With trocar injuries most surgeons would feel most comfortable converting the procedure to open laparotomy and exploring and performing the intra-peritoneal repair under direct vision.

When a trocar causes a retroperitoneal injury and hematoma, the injured site must be explored and usually repair of a major vessel is required. A case report of a trocar injury to a major vessel and review of the literature in 1988 cited 15 similar cases.[10] Most injuries were related to insertion of the Veress needle and only two were caused by trocars. The aorta and iliac vessels were the most commonly injured vessels, and recovery after simple suture was the rule. Two of 15 patients died.

One survey showed that only 50% of Veress needle injuries required surgical repair.[13] The researchers found that because the puncture wound created by a Veress needle is of such small diameter, most needle puncture wounds in a vessel or bowel heal spontaneously.

Since the great demand for laparoscopy began in 1989, more surgeons with minimal experience are performing laparoscopy. Although safety features have been incorporated into the design of disposable trocars and needles, the geometric increase in the frequency of their use has probably made vascular and bowel complications no less common. There is a pervasive feeling that these injuries occur much more often and are underreported. However, in a recent study by Airan,[15] a questionnaire was sent to 4300 surgical department chairmen in the United States. There were 1200 replies, which reported data on 27,204 laparoscopic operations performed by 2386 surgeons. The complication rate was 1.5%. The most frequent complications were vascular injuries and intraoperative bleeding (114), which required conversion to open laparotomy. Injury to the aorta, vena cava, or iliac vessels occurred in 12 patients. Forty bowel injuries were reported, including stomach (2), duodenum (8), small intestine (17), and colon (13). Fifteen deaths were reported.

Prevention

Although these injuries can never be completely prevented, their incidence can be kept low. In an effort to prevent such injuries, disposable trocars have been redesigned to include a safety shield that advances over the trocar after the peritoneal cavity has been entered (Fig. 9-1). One must keep in mind, however, that the safety shield does not eliminate trocar injuries and is no substitute for careful technique. No studies comparing disposable vs. nondisposable trocars have yet been performed, but I suspect in terms of safety the differences are few. In fact, the incidence of trocar and needle injuries in 250,000 laparoscopic procedures performed with nondisposable trocars was no higher than that in a series in which disposable trocars were used.[6,15]

In addition to using trocars with safety shields, practicing the following maneuvers can limit the risk of injury: (1) creating an adequate skin incision that will accommodate the trocar so that undue force is not needed to penetrate the skin and subcutaneous tissue; (2) clearing the subcutaneous tissue to allow the needle to abut directly onto the fascia, where it will penetrate the fascia more easily; (3) checking that there is full pneumoperitoneum before puncturing the fascia with the needle and trocars; (4) checking that the safety shield will function properly prior to use of the trocar; and (5) directing the angle of trocar to the pelvis with a gentle and steady pushing motion and then angling the trocar upward toward the abdominal wall after it pierces the peritoneum.

Finally, it should be remembered that open laparoscopy offers the chance to directly place a sheath or port without risk of trocar injury. Some surgeons routinely opt for open laparoscopy when placing the umbilical port, whereas others use it selectively, employing it when adhesions or scars are present in the lower abdomen. Once the surgeon has examined the peritoneal cavity through the camera in the umbilical port, the surgeon, guided by the camera, can place the other ports. Open laparoscopy has a clear, definite, and expanding role and should be 100% safe. Clearly the greatest risk of trocar injury lies with the initial trocar puncture. The risk is significantly less with the subsequent placement of the remaining ports, since they are not inserted blindly.

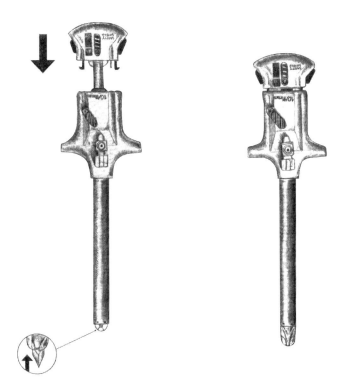

FIGURE 9-1 • The safety shield of the trocar should be checked to be certain it is functioning properly. The handle of the trocar should be engaged just prior to its insertion into the abdomen. Checking that the instrument is functional will limit the force applied to the abdomen and therefore prevent injury to underlying viscera.

COMPLICATIONS OF INSUFFLATION

When pneumoperitoneum is achieved with insufflation, the increased intra-abdominal pressure and the use of gases that are absorbed into the bloodstream cause physiologic changes.[4,16-18] Elevating intra-abdominal pressures to 10 to 15 mm Hg causes a systemic rise in venous and arterial pressures. EKG changes secondary to diaphragmatic displacement may occur. Carbon dioxide also causes a rise in blood pressure (a sympathetic response to hypercarbia). When intra-abdominal pressure exceeds 20 mm Hg, cardiac output decreases, as does venous return. Arrhythmias are not uncommon. Blood gases are also altered with carbon dioxide. They include a fall in arterial pH, an increase in Pco_2 and a decrease in Po_2. Many of these fluctuations are self-corrected when the patient is under general anesthesia and on a ventilator.

A less serious complication of insufflation is extravasation of infused gas into the omentum, mesentery, or preperitoneal space.[19] Mediastinal emphysema due to the injection of carbon dioxide between the peritoneum and fascia is usually self-limiting. Dissection to the neck is sometimes noted but generally requires no treatment. Maneuvers that confirm correct placement of the needle are effective in preventing this complication (see Chapter 2). High insufflation pressures with low flow generally indicate malposition of the needle or obstruction to outflow from the insufflator.

Gas Embolization

The fear when using any gas for insufflation is its absorption into the bloodstream in sufficient quantities to cause embolization. Fortunately, this complication is extremely rare: 1 in every 65,000 laparoscopic cases. Because carbon dioxide offers the lowest risk of embolization, it is the gas used most often for insufflation. A volume of carbon dioxide greater than 1 L must be injected intravascularly before cardiac output falls significantly. The mechanism of decreased cardiac output is secondary to right ventricular obstruction from the gas. Carbon dioxide enters the venous system by direct absorption under increased intra-abdominal pressure or by direct access to a vein that has been opened directly during operative dissection. When gas embolization is recognized, insufflation must be ceased immediately and all carbon dioxide in the abdominal cavity must be released through the instrument ports.

If cardiovascular collapse occurs, in rare instances it may be due to a profound vasovagal response.[20] Another cause of cardiovascular collapse is the impaired venous return from a carbon dioxide embolus in the venous system. In the latter situation, appropriate treatment measures include maintaining cardiovascular stability, placing the patient supine, and rapidly evacuating carbon dioxide from the peritoneal cavity. At times hyperbaric oxygen has been used.[16,21-23]

INFREQUENT COMPLICATIONS

As with open procedures, wound infections or hematomas may occur but are extremely rare (3 per 1000 laparoscopic procedures).[16] They occur in the tract through which the gallbladder has been removed. Rarely, infections may be secondary to subcuticular suture materials. Hematomas at the site of trocar punctures are usually of little clinical significance and absorb spontaneously.

When the 5 and 10 mm ports are withdrawn, omentum or bowel may be caught in the fascial puncture site. If the bowel stays trapped in the fascia beneath the skin, this situation may not be recognized until intestinal necrosis and peritonitis occur. This occurrence is extremely rare.[24,25] It can be avoided by palpating the fascial opening with the tip of a hemostat before closing the subcuticular tissues.

Even more uncommon is the tracking and implanting of malignant cells into a port puncture wound. The development of a metastatic nodule has been reported in this situation.[26] It is, however, no different from malignant implantation into a scar during open laparotomy.

Dissection of blood to a preexisting hernia sac may make it look as if the patient has a tender symptomatic inguinal hernia, but this, too, is an uncommon complication.

OPERATIVE COMPLICATIONS

Complications encountered or created during the cholecystectomy itself are identical to those sustained during open cholecystectomy, namely, electrocautery and laser injuries, bleeding, bile leaks, common duct injuries, liver laceration, and subhepatic collections of bile or blood.

Electrosurgery and Laser Injuries

As familiar as surgeons are with electrosurgery, bowel injuries have been reported with its use.[27] If recognized during laparoscopy, these injuries can be repaired. Unfortunately, the area of burn, necrosis, and perforation may not be apparent until several days postoperatively when sepsis has occurred. Rarely, death has been reported due to sepsis from a bowel perforation.[27] With electrosurgery, the energy is conducted through the patient to the grounding pad. The dispersed energy varies with the strength of the current. The concern that electrical energy might cause injury during closed laparotomy has been raised. At least 12 cases of intestinal perforation discovered after the use of electrosurgery have been reported.[27] Histologic examinations questioned whether the injuries were the result of intraoperative mechanical trauma or electrical burns. Nevertheless, the safety record with monopolar electrosurgery is enviable, considering how frequently it is used. For safety purposes the lowest effective current level should be used, keeping in mind the energy of cutting current is 10 times less than that of coagulation current. Current conducted through plastic sheaths may cause thermal injury to viscera.

Laser injuries may be incurred by the operator or the patient. The risk of eye injury is minimized with the use of protective goggles. Bowel and vascular injuries to the patient can occur as with electrosurgery.[28] However, the penetration depth offered by laser is more precise.

Bile Fistulas

In the difficult gallbladder the appearance of bile in the drain heralds this complication. If the abdomen is not drained postoperatively, abdominal distention or leakage of bile through a port site suggests that a bile fistula has developed. Bile drainage may occur immediately after the procedure or days later. If the leakage originates from the cystic duct, lateral common duct, right posterior hepatic duct, or liver bed (from an accessory bile duct), it will stop spontaneously. The time it takes for spontaneous closure to occur is dependent on the pressure gradient between the bile duct and duodenum and the size of the defect. Whatever the source, a drain should be percutaneously placed as guided by fluoroscopy, ultrasonography, or CT. Injection of contrast will usually not initially fill the duct system or identify the site of leakage. After 1 week, the cavity will diminish in size, and a repeat study will demonstrate the site of the defect. When the drain is positioned in the subhepatic space, gravity drainage to a leg bag can be implemented and the daily amount of drainage recorded. If drainage is more than 600 cc per day and the cystic duct or the common duct is leaking, an endoscopic stent may also be inserted to occlude the opening in the duct. Patients may be followed up on an outpatient basis until the fistula has closed.

Complete transections of a major duct must be surgically repaired. Since a decompressed, nonobstructed duct is thin walled and of small diameter, a complete transection is difficult to repair. The use of a roux or interposed limb is my preferred method for reanastomosing the duct. The patient should be advised of the possibility of stricture development. Injury to a segmental duct will usually stricture and does not require repair.

PROBLEMS AND SOLUTIONS

Case 1

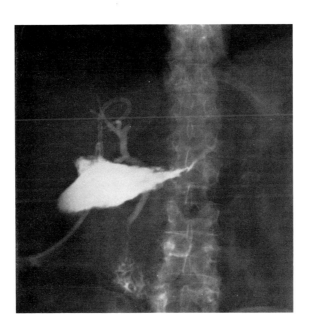

In this patient a delayed bile leak from the cystic duct was detected. Bile drainage from a port wound suggested that this complication was present. The site of the leakage—the cystic duct—closed spontaneously.

In some cases leakage of bile is due to malocclusion of the clip. Therefore its proper application should be verified visually to be certain that the clip has not "scissored" and that the duct is closed.

Common Duct Injury

The most serious complication in laparoscopic cholecystectomy is injury to the common hepatic duct or right hepatic duct. Since this complication can also happen with open cholecystectomy, its occurrence will not be eliminated by the new methodology.

The first step in avoiding injury to the common duct is to be aware of the anatomic situation, particularly as it relates to the cystic duct–common duct junction. In this respect a cholangiogram helps define aberrant anatomy prior to transection of any structure. However, it is not a substitute for visualizing the cystic duct–common duct junction.

At some hospitals, obtaining a cholangiogram is not as easy as it should be because technicians are unavailable, there is equipment malfunction, cannulation is difficult because the cystic duct is small or obstructed by stones, or, despite repeated studies, visualization of the ducts remains poor. If an adequate cholangiogram cannot be obtained and if the duct anatomy is uncertain, the following steps must be followed if laparoscopic cholecystectomy is to be continued. The cystic duct–common duct junction and the common hepatic duct above and below the cystic duct must be identified. This basic tenet of open cholecystectomy holds true for laparoscopic cholecystectomy as well. During laparoscopic cholecystectomy, the common duct is tented by traction with the infundibular port clamp. For this reason, the lower third of the bile duct appears as a continuation of the cystic duct.[29] Thus the visual impression of a very long cystic duct given by this en face view is incorrect and misleading. Since the eye (the camera) is beneath the hilum and parallel to the common duct, the view of the cystic duct–common duct junction is head on. Depth perception above the cystic duct is very poor. The lack of liver retraction gives the impression that the cystic duct is almost contiguous with the hilum. Very little of the common hepatic duct is seen with the camera at the umbilicus. An aberrant or low insertion of a right hepatic duct is of particular concern. I always place a spatula behind the cystic duct and follow the cystic duct to its junction with the common duct. The hepatic duct above the cystic duct must also be visualized. Replacing clamps and maneuvering the cystic duct may expose the hepatic duct. If this maneuver fails, the laparoscope and camera should be moved to the fundic port, where the 5 mm port should be replaced with a 10 mm sheath. The view will then be head on to the common hepatic duct (see Chapter 4).

When acute cholecystitis distorts or retracts the hilar structures or makes dissection otherwise difficult, the surgeon's eye (with the camera at the umbilicus) is at the wrong level. In this circumstance, the gallbladder should be dissected retrograde from fundus to hilum. Although many believe this is not possible or safe laparoscopically, the opposite is true (see Chapter 5). Retrograde dissection is done by first decompressing the gallbladder if it is acutely distended. The fundus is then pulled from the liver, and countertraction is provided by exposing the liver at the gallbladder–liver bed junction with a second clamp. The plane between liver and gallbladder is entered with a dissecting instrument and the gallbladder is dissected retrograde. If this approach fails to provide adequate exposure of the cystic duct–common duct junction, at this point it is safer to convert to an open cholecystectomy.

PROBLEMS AND SOLUTIONS

Case 2

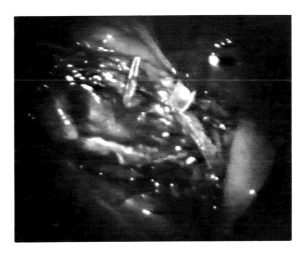

In this patient, the infundibulum of the gallbladder and cystic duct were so tenuous and necrotic that dissection with the spatula caused a tear in the cystic duct, which was identified. The gallbladder was completely freed from the liver bed and then the cystic duct was grasped and dissected to the common duct, where it was secured with an EndoLoop.

Gallstones in the Peritoneal Cavity

At times, stones fall from the gallbladder through the cystic duct or through openings in the gallbladder wall. These openings are iatrogenic or spontaneous. Perforations are unselective in that both bile and stones exit the gallbladder. The stones and bile usually remain in the subhepatic space above the transverse colon. When gallstones fall from the gallbladder, the gallbladder dissection is completed and bile is suctioned from the subhepatic space. The stones are exposed in a cluster and may be retrieved in clamps and placed in drains, gloves, or stone bags. Single stones may be removed directly.

Stones left in the peritoneal cavity cause little harm. Isolated reports of stone migration into bowel, kidney, and bladder have appeared in the literature.[30] If the stones are calcified, there is greater concern since these stones will show on a flat-plate roentgenogram of the abdomen. While these fallen stones should not be a problem, the situation has medicolegal implications in some patients.

PROBLEMS AND SOLUTIONS

Case 3

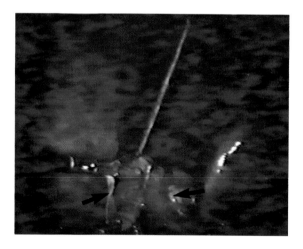

The gallbladder (right arrow), having been freed from the liver, was placed into a 1-inch Penrose drain held open by clamps (left arrow) placed through the infundibular port and the fundic port.

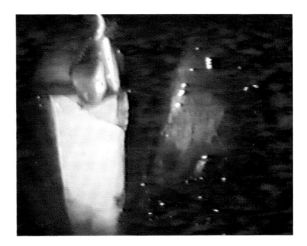

The stones that fell from the gallbladder as it separated from the liver were placed in the Penrose drain together with the gallbladder and removed. The bottom of the drain was tied off.

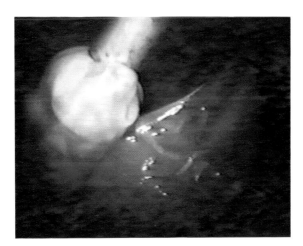

The drain has been closed and drawn into the operating port, where it was removed with the sheath.

Case 4

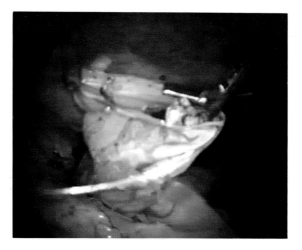

The gangrenous gallbladder and stones were removed from the liver bed. Because it was so thick and necrotic, the gallbladder along with the stones were placed in a prototype stone bag with a nylon drawstring.

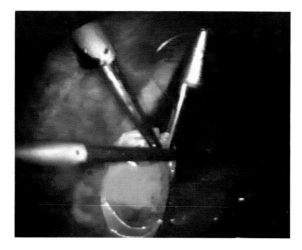

The gallbladder and stones have been secured and the strings are drawn closed.

Case 5

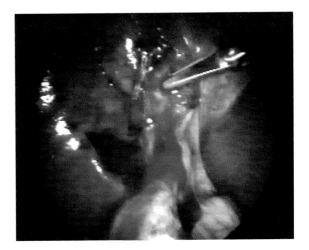

The scissors point to a large impacted calculus in the cystic duct. It was removed to facilitate dissection and ligation of the cystic duct.

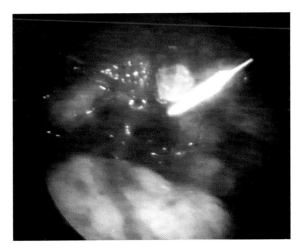

The cystic duct was opened by a spatulated cautery, and the stone was milked out with the scissors. The stone was delivered through the operating port with 5 mm claw forceps.

Case 6

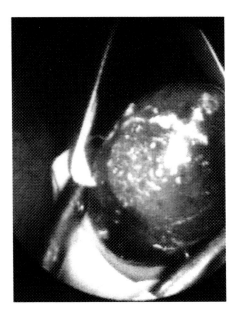

A large stone fell from the gallbladder between the liver and abdominal wall as the gallbladder was pulled through the abdominal wall. It was retrieved and placed in a Penrose drain.

Bleeding From the Liver Bed

When the gallbladder mesentery is inflamed or obliterated because of cholecystitis, bleeding may occur from the liver bed. When this happens, it is easier to first complete the dissection of the gallbladder from the liver bed and place the gallbladder between the liver and lateral abdominal wall. Grasping clamps are then used to expose the gallbladder fossa. A 28 Fr chest tube placed on a 5 mm irrigation probe increases flow and suction capabilities. The liver bed is irrigated, and bleeding points are identified and coagulated. Bleeding from a liver laceration is usually caused by a penetrating scissors injury or an overzealous insertion of the port. Bleeding from the liver bed stops spontaneously or with direct pressure and rarely requires suturing or an omental pack.

PROBLEMS AND SOLUTIONS

Case 7

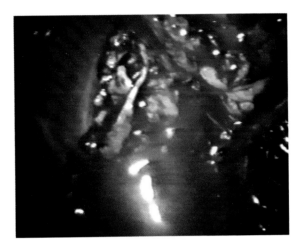

Bleeding from the liver can be seen. A gangrenous gallbladder was dissected in this patient who had multiple previous operations. Although the main artery was ligated, a posterior segmental branch bled in the liver bed.

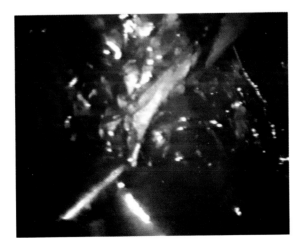

The vessel has been clamped.

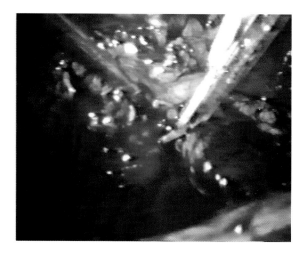

Once the bleeding was controlled, a clip was applied to the vessel.

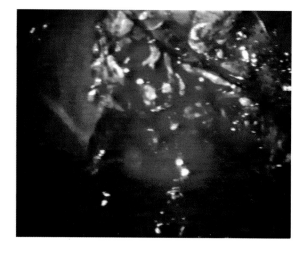

A clamp has been applied to the upper end of the vessel and bleeding is completely controlled.

Case 8

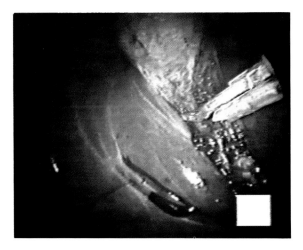

A small posterior divisional branch of the cystic artery was identified in the bed of the liver and then clipped and divided.

Cystic Artery Bleeding

In the course of dissection in both open and laparoscopic cholecystectomy, bleeding from a divisional branch of a cystic artery sometimes occurs. When the cystic artery is injured, the following steps should be taken. The instrument that caused the injury should be used to apply pressure directly to the bleeding vessel. Extravasated blood should be suctioned. At the same time the laparoscope should be backed into its sheath so blood will not obscure the tip of the laparoscope and blur vision. After a few minutes, pressure can be lightened and the offending vessel usually can be seen and clipped. If the bleeding is brisk and instrument pressure does not control it, the vessel should be clamped. A clip can then be applied to the vessel. The advantage of video magnification in this situation is most apparent.

PROBLEMS AND SOLUTIONS

Case 9

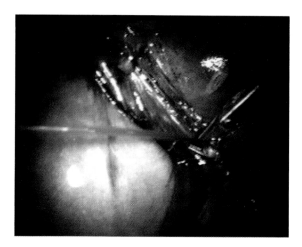

During this operation, transection of the cystic duct was followed by an unanticipated surprise. The scissors transected the cystic artery, which lay just posterior to the cystic duct. A stream of blood is seen directed to the left and the clipped proximal cystic duct is seen beneath the scissors.

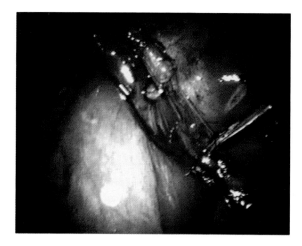

The scissors were used to compress the artery. Blood in the area was suctioned.

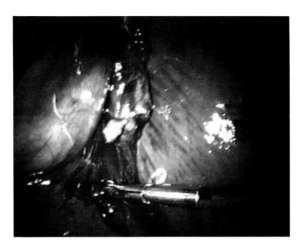

Despite pressure being applied for several minutes, the bleeding would not stop spontaneously. The end of the artery was then grasped by a clamp, which controlled the bleeding.

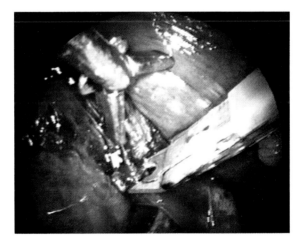

After the clamp was removed, the bleeding did not resume. The vessel was then secured by a clip. A needle holder introduced through the infundibular port was poised if bleeding persisted.

Case 10

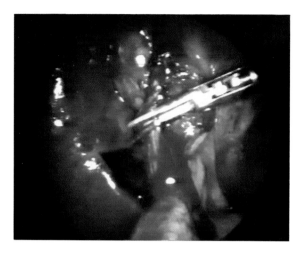

A small anterior divisional branch of the cystic artery next to the cystic duct was identified. It has been clipped and divided with scissors.

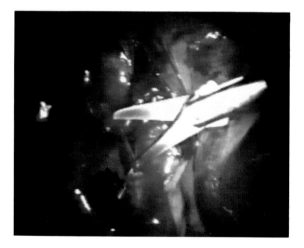

In the process of dissecting the artery from the duct, the clip was dislodged (arrow) and a stream of blood from the artery directed toward the hilum was seen.

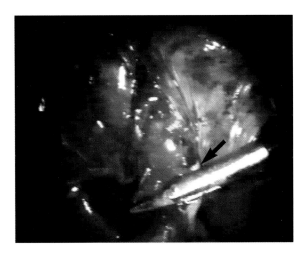

To control the bleeding, the vessel (arrow) was compressed with the scissors and blood was aspirated from the area.

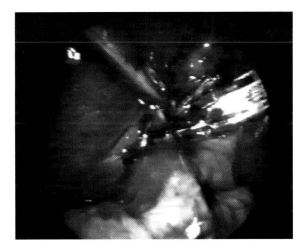

Despite compression for several minutes, release of pressure was followed by resumption of bleeding. Therefore the infundibular port clamp was used to grab the end of the bleeding vessel and a clip was placed beneath it. Care was taken to maintain an appropriate distance between the end of the vessel and the common duct.

REFERENCES

1. Carmichael DE. Laparoscopy: Cardiac considerations. Fertil Steril 22:69-70, 1971.
2. Scott DB, Julian DG. Observations on cardiac arrhythmias during laparoscopy. Br Med J 1:411-413, 1972.
3. Hamilton WK, McDonald JS, Fischer HW, et al. Postoperative respiratory complications. Anesthesiology 25:607-612, 1964.
4. Versichelen L, Serryn R, Rolly G, et al. Physiopathologic changes during anesthesia administration for gynecologic laparoscopy. J Reprod Med 29:697-700, 1984.
5. Roberts CJ, Goodman NW. Gastroesophageal reflux during elective laparoscopy. Anaesthesia 45:1009-1011, 1990.
6. Riedel HH, Willenbrock-Lehmann E, Mecke H, et al. The frequency of distribution of various pelviscopic (laparoscopic) operations, including complication rates—Statistics of the Federal Republic of Germany in the years 1983-1985. Zentralbl Gynakol 111:78-91, 1989.
7. Katz M, Beck P, Tancer ML. Major vessel injury during laparoscopy: Anatomy of two cases. Am J Obstet Gynecol 135:544-545, 1979.
8. Mintz M. Risks and prophylaxis in laparoscopy: A survey of 100,000 cases. J Reprod Med 18:269-272, 1977.
9. Lynn SC, Katz AR, Ross PJ. Aortic perforation sustained at laparoscopy. J Reprod Med 27:217-219, 1982.
10. Baadsgaard SE, Bille S, Egeblad K. Major vascular injury during gynecologic laparoscopy: Report of two cases and review of published cases. Acta Obstet Gynecol Scand 68:283-285, 1988.
11. Peterson HB, Greenspan JR, Ory HW. Death following puncture of the aorta during laparoscopic sterilization. Obstet Gynecol 59:133-134, 1982.
12. Shin CS. Vascular injury secondary to laparoscopy. NY State J Med 82:935-936, 1982.
13. Yuzpe AA. Pneumoperitoneum needle and trocar injuries in laparoscopy: A survey on possible contributing factors and prevention. J Reprod Med 35(5):485-490, 1990.
14. Reich H, McGlynn F. Laparoscopic repair of bladder injury. Obstet Gynecol 76:909-910, 1990.
15. Airan MA. Report on presentation at the Society of American Gastrointestinal Endoscopic Surgeons. Gen Surg News, July 1991; personal communication, August 1991.
16. Bailey RW. Complications of laparoscopic general surgery. In Zucker KA, ed. Surgical Laparoscopy. St. Louis: Quality Medical Publishing, 1991, pp 311-342.
17. Marshall RL, Jebson PJR, Davie IT, et al. Circulatory effects of carbon dioxide insufflation of the peritoneal cavity for laparoscopy. Br J Anaesth 44:680-684, 1972.
18. Lenz RJ, Thomas TA, Wilkins DG. Cardiovascular changes during laparoscopy: Studies of stroke volume and cardiac output using impedance cardiography. Anaesthesia 31:4-12, 1976.
19. Kalhan SB, Reaney JA, Collins RL. Pneumomediastinum and subcutaneous emphysema during laparoscopy. Cleve Clin J Med 57(7):639-642, 1990.

20. DePlater RMH, Jones ISC. Non-fatal carbon dioxide embolism during laparoscopy. Anaesth Intensive Care 17:359-361, 1989.
21. Gomar C, Fernandez C, Villalonga A, et al. Carbon dioxide embolism during laparoscopy and hysteroscopy. Ann Fr Anesth Reanim 4:380-382, 1985.
22. Brantley JC III, Riley PM. Cardiovascular collapse during laparoscope: A report of two cases. Am J Obstet Gynecol 159:735-737, 1988.
23. McGrath BJ, Zimmerman JE, Williams JF, et al. Carbon dioxide embolism treated with hyperbaric oxygen. Can J Anaesth 36(5):586-589, 1989.
24. Thomas AG, McLymont F, Moshipur J. Incarcerated hernia after laparoscopic sterilization: A case report. J Reprod Med 35(6):639-640, 1990.
25. Kiilholma P, Mlakinen J. Incarcerated Richter's hernia after laparoscopy: A case report. Eur J Obstet Gynecol Reprod Biol 28(1):75-77, 1988.
26. Miralles RM, Petit J, Ginle L, et al. Metastatic cancer spread at the laparoscopic puncture site: Report of a case in a patient with carcinoma of the ovary. A case report. Eur J Gynaecol Oncol 10(6):442-444, 1989.
27. Soderstrom RM, Levy BS. Bowel injuries during laparoscopy: Causes and medicolegal questions. Continuing Obstet Gynecol 27:41-45, 1986.
28. Hertzmann P. Thermal instrumentation for laparoscopic general surgical procedures. In Zucker KA, ed. Surgical Laparoscopy. St. Louis: Quality Medical Publishing, 1991, pp 57-75.
29. Cooperman AM. Technical tips for laparoscopic cholecystectomy. J Laparoendosc Surg 3(2), 1991.
30. Cooperman AM, Dickson ER, ReMine WH. Changing concepts in the surgical treatment of gallstone ileus: A review of 15 cases with emphasis on diagnosis and treatment. Ann Surg 167:377-383, 1968.

• Invited Commentary •

As the initial wave of enthusiasm for laparoscopic surgery has reached the shores of surgical practice, Dr. Cooperman's reassessment of technology-related complications is appropriate.

Although laparoscopic cholecystectomy was introduced as a laser procedure, electrosurgery is now recognized as the preferred energy source for tissue dissection because of efficacy and cost. Laser and electrosurgery are equally safe, but insulation failure and capacitive coupling may lead to injuries with radio frequency electrical energy. Both of these problems have now been resolved by the addition of an electrical shield (Electroscope) that collects the energy of capacitive coupling and dynamically monitors for fault conditions. Another potentially dangerous aspect of laparoscopic electrosurgical dissection is the unintended transfer of electrical energy by direct contact of the activated electrode to other metal equipment (graspers or laparoscope) within the abdomen, resulting in the unrecognized transfer of stray energy to the bowel, out of the view of the laparoscope. The use of all-metal cannulas greatly reduces the chance of injury to the bowel by dispersing any stray energy at the abdominal wall.

Although 90% of surgeons still use the expensive disposable trocar/cannula with the "safety shield," it is my strong opinion that the "safety shield" does not confer safety to the experienced surgeon or the patient and indeed may be a misnomer.[1] In a recent audit of our first 1000 cases, the only bowel perforation occurred in the 1% of patients in whom a disposable trocar/cannula was used. In an effort to limit the amount of force required to introduce the trocar/cannula, the umbilical fascia can be incised directly with a knife blade. Oftentimes, a peritoneal defect can be visualized, allowing direct insertion of the trocar/cannula prior to insufflation. Use of the all-plastic cannulas and particularly the hybrid metal/plastic cannulas increases the risk of inadvertent electrical burn to the bowel in certain scenarios and poses environmental hazards.

Although surgeons always have argued the merits of various techniques, there is little argument regarding the most effective way to deal with common bile duct injury: prevention. The safety net is laparotomy prior to complications.

As fiscally responsible surgeons, we must be increasingly cognizant of the cost of technologic choices and the interface between science, commerce, education, and patient care.

C. Randle Voyles, M.D., M.S.

Associate Clinical Professor,
Department of Surgery,
University of Mississippi,
Jackson, Miss.

REFERENCE

1. Voyles CR, Petro AB, Meena AL, et al. A practical approach to laparoscopic cholecystectomy. Am J Surg 161:365-370, 1991.

• Invited Commentary •

Dr. Cooperman presents an excellent summary of complications encountered during therapeutic laparoscopy. For the most part, I concur wholeheartedly with his approach. I would include pregnancy as a general risk factor. Many now believe that with adequate monitoring of the fetus, laparoscopic cholecystectomy can be safely performed in the pregnant patient, especially if the operation is performed during that window of time after the first trimester so that teratogenic effects can be avoided but before 20 weeks' gestation when the uterus begins to enlarge above the umbilicus.

I concur that trocar and needle injuries are certainly underreported as they tend to occur as isolated incidents in individual surgeon's experiences and thus are not commonly published. I support the wider use of the open technique for initial peritoneal penetration because it virtually eliminates the most feared complication of laparoscopy—major vessel injury.

Gas embolization is a complication that fortunately I have not had to deal with. However, in addition to the maneuvers described by Dr. Cooperman, I would place the patient in the Trendelenburg position to try to move the gas out of the pulmonary outflow tract.

Abdominal wall hematoma is a complication that can be a source of considerable pain for the patient and, when the patient's blood count drops in the postoperative period, a diagnostic dilemma for the surgeon. It is important that this complication be differentiated from intra-abdominal bleeding. Treatment of abdominal wall hematomas is largely supportive because in most cases they resolve spontaneously. Rarely is exploration of the hematoma with ligation of the bleeding vessel required.

Our approach to bleeding from the cystic artery is slightly different from that of Dr. Cooperman. We have found that most bleeding can be controlled by blind but gentle application of atraumatic grasping forceps, which cannot damage critical structures in the porta hepatis. The abdomen can then be thoroughly suctioned and irrigated and the offending vessel carefully isolated and controlled.

The loss of gallstones into the peritoneal cavity is inevitable in some laparoscopic cholecystectomy patients. Results of studies in rabbits in our laboratory suggest that bilirubinate stones will commonly resorb and cholesterol stones will persist. However, we noted surprisingly little inflammation around the stones. Every attempt should be made to remove lost gallstones but certainly this should not be the sole criterion for conversion to open cholecystectomy.

The final issue is that of common bile duct injury. Dr. Cooperman's excellent suggestions should be heeded. I plan to incorporate movement of the camera to ancillary ports into my technique. We believe that the most dangerous anatomic situation in laparoscopic cholecystectomy exists with acute, subacute, or chronic inflammation, resulting in the cystic duct being fibrosed into the infundibulum of the gallbladder, making it, for all practical purposes, absent. Traction to the right makes the distal common bile duct appear to be the cystic duct, exiting the gallbladder. Thus we exercise extreme caution when dealing with the infundibulum of the gallbladder when chronic scarring or inflammation is involved.

Robert J. Fitzgibbons, Jr., M.D., F.A.C.S.

Associate Professor of Surgery,
Chief, Division of General Surgery,
Department of Surgery, Creighton University,
School of Medicine,
Omaha, Neb.

·10·

Outcome

The aphorism about surgical operations—Those who have enthusiasm have no controls, and those who have controls have no enthusiasm[1]—will not be applied to clinical research on laparoscopic cholecystectomy. The protagonists of laparoscopic cholecystectomy are satisfied patients who have had successful surgery. Subjectively, they number in the thousands. Objectively, reports of experiences with large numbers of these patients are just now being published.[2-8] These reports attempt to deal with bottom-line issues: Is laparoscopic cholecystectomy safe? What are the risks? What is the conversion rate to open cholecystectomy? How often are common duct stones found? These questions have been difficult to address because until now most reports reflect early and limited operative experiences with small numbers of patients and liberal exclusion of certain patients (patient bias). There has also been a suspicion that only the best results were being reported and the less than optimal results were not published.

RECOVERY

The short hospital stay and early return to full activity after laparoscopic cholecystectomy have been confirmed in reports and universally acclaimed by surgeons. A survey of 104 French patients and 84 American patients after laparoscopic cholecystectomy revealed postoperative discomfort resolved completely in 73% of French and 93% of American patients within 10 days.[9] All but 16 patients returned to normal social activities within 2 weeks after surgery. The statistics regarding return to work were equally impressive: 63% of American and 25% of French patients returned to work within 2 weeks, while 14% of American and 30% of French patients required a convalescence of at least 1 month after surgery. Several patients had returned to heavy physical work within 1 week after surgery. There was a correlation between the type of work and length of convalescence. The authors suggest that return to work is influenced as much by cultural habits as by physical disability. Because this was a small study, inferences between patients in different countries cannot really be made. However, it is clear that many patients are physically able to return to work soon after laparoscopic surgery.

Many patients do not require hospitalization at all after laparoscopic cholecystectomy for chronic cholecystitis. An overnight stay is often a matter of patient preference. Spaw, Reddick, and Olsen[10] noted that up to 20% of recent operations they performed were done on an ambulatory basis. Of the first 25 patients on whom I performed laparoscopic cholecystectomy, nine (36%) were treated on an ambulatory basis and seven others (35%) were operated on late in the day and remained hospitalized less than 15 hours.[11] I have found that approximately 75% of chronic cholecystitis patients can be treated on an ambulatory basis. These patients, however, are cautioned to call or return to the hospital if there is excess pain or if concern is otherwise raised. They must live close enough to the hospital so that the patient, family, and physician are comfortable with the decision to proceed with treatment on an ambulatory basis. The patient is contacted the morning following hospital discharge to make sure all is well.

The length of hospitalization unfortunately is often determined by many hospitals on the basis of reimbursement. This is balanced by the desire of insurance carriers to have as many procedures as possible performed on an ambulatory basis. Both views are understandable but they may be contrary to the health interests of many patients. These issues will be worked out with time and experience.

MORTALITY

Deaths associated with laparoscopic cholecystectomy are rare but have been reported. A review of a European experience[2] (1236 patients, 20 surgeons, 0 deaths), the Southern Surgeons Club study[5] (1518 patients, 59 surgeons, one death), and the Society of American Gastrointestinal Endoscopic Surgeons (SAGES) questionnaire survey[6] (27,204 patients, 2300 surgeons, 15 deaths [0.05%]) confirm the statistical safety of laparoscopic cholecystectomy.

In the SAGES study, of the 15 deaths, two were due to bile duct injury, two to pulmonary embolus, and one each to duodenal injury, colon injury, small bowel injury, cystic duct injury, aortic injury, and caval injury. One patient died of a myocardial infarction and one from pneumonia. One death was due to ischemic bowel and one to necrotizing fasciitis. One patient presented to an emergency room several days postoperatively and died from an undetermined cause. The data presented in the SAGES study are valuable in that they reflect the initial experience of most respondents. (The average number of cases performed by the respondents was <10.) Most deaths and complications occur early in a surgeon's experience with laparoscopic cholecystectomy, and the incidence decreases with experience. If the SAGES statistics are an accurate representation of the surgeon's early experience, laparoscopic cholecystectomy has an acceptable procedure-related mortality rate that will continue to fall as expertise is gained. Although the mortality rate is low, it is probably higher than that for comparable young patients undergoing elective open cholecystectomy for chronic cholecystitis. For chronic cholecystitis, a rare cause of death is the open cholecystectomy itself.

MORBIDITY
Bile Duct Injury

The most feared complication of laparoscopic cholecystectomy is bile duct injury. In the European experience, bile duct injury occurred in four of 1203 patients.[2] In the Southern Surgeons Club study,[5] bile duct injury was recognized at laparoscopy in seven patients and was corrected by open laparotomy. Three other such injuries were recognized on postoperative days 3, 5, and 14, respectively. Five of the seven bile duct injuries occurred before the 13th operation; the other two occurred in the 25th and 43rd procedures. After the first 13 procedures, the incidence of duct injuries fell to 0.1%.

In the SAGES study,[6] common duct injuries were reported in 99 patients, 84 of whom required open surgery for repair. Eighty-one other patients had delayed bile leaks: 49 were treated surgically and 33 were treated by percutaneous drainage or observation.

My impression is that bile leakage, bleeding, and common duct injuries are more common with laparoscopic cholecystectomy than with open cholecystectomy, particularly when laparoscopic surgery programs are first initiated. Most laparoscopic cholecystectomies are done for chronic cholecystitis; for the more difficult gallbladders, the incidence of bile duct injuries could be higher. These complications occur significantly more often following laparoscopic cholecystectomy than after open cholecystectomy. The incidence will decrease with time, improved instrumentation, and increased experience.

Common Duct Stones

Since common duct stones have a natural history often marked by a long quiescent period, their exact incidence at laparoscopic cholecystectomy would only be known if there were a long follow-up period or if intraoperative cholangiograms were routinely obtained. In most series, intraoperative cholangiograms are obtained selectively. In the Southern Surgeons Club experience,[5] less than 2% of patients had proven or suspected common duct stones. This incidence is at least 8% less than predicted since cholangiography was selectively performed. The series will bear further follow-up. A report of 53 cholangiograms in 58 patients undergoing laparoscopic cholecystectomy detected common duct stones in six patients: in five the finding was unsuspected.[12]

The incidence of common duct stones does not vary between laparoscopic cholecystectomy and open cholecystectomy because common duct stones are a reflection of the disease, not its treatment.[12]

Vascular and Bowel Injuries

In the SAGES questionnaire by Airan,[6] vascular injuries and significant intraoperative bleeding were the most common complications. Major vessel injury to the aorta, inferior vena cava, or iliac vessels occurred in 12 patients and 57 patients suffered injury to the portal vessels. Bleeding from the gallbladder bed complicated 31 cases, and 18 other patients had delayed bleeding, 12 of whom required surgery to control the hemorrhage.

Forty bowel injuries were noted. Two were gastric, 8 were duodenal, 17 were small intestine, and 13 were colonic. Laparotomy was required in 35. These numbers reaffirm an acceptable morbidity.

CONVERSION TO OPEN CHOLECYSTECTOMY

The conversion rate to open cholecystectomy varies depending on the surgeon's experience, operative finding, and indication for surgery (acute vs. chronic cholecystitis). Surgeons experienced in laparoscopic cholecystectomy indicate a low rate of complications and a low incidence of conversion to open cholecystectomy.[10,13-16] When consecutive unselected patients underwent laparoscopic cholecystectomy, less than 3% of patients required conversion to open cholecystectomy and significant complications occurred in less than 2%.[14]

COST

The assumption that laparoscopic cholecystectomy is less expensive than standard open cholecystectomy has not been clearly substantiated. The shorter hospital stay must be balanced against the increased operating room costs (lasers, disposable ports, and instruments) and longer operative time.

A cost savings favoring laparoscopic cholecystectomy over open cholecystectomy was noted in a comparative study from Ohio.[17] In a study from Mississippi in which electrosurgery rather than laser was used and nondisposable instruments and selective cholangiography were implemented, the average cost of laparoscopic cholecystectomy was again less than that of open cholecystectomy.[4] The cost of laparoscopic cholecystectomy varies among New York hospitals, but it is certainly higher than in Ohio and Mississippi. The ambulatory reimbursement rate for laparoscopic cholecystectomy in our small New York hospital is approximately $2000.

CLINICAL EXPERIENCE

My personal experience involves 300 consecutive cholecystectomy patients. The only selection criteria were that the patients have symptomatic gallbladder disease and be able to tolerate an anesthetic and laparoscopy. The first 25 patients included 13 with chronic cholecystitis, seven with acute cholecystitis, two with cirrhosis, and three with subacute cholecystitis (recent history of an acute attack with chronic cholecystitis). Nine patients were treated on an ambulatory basis, seven were operated on late in the day and were hospitalized for less than 15 hours, seven were hospitalized for 1 day, and two patients remained hospitalized for 24 to 48 hours. The operative time averaged 50 minutes (range, 25 to 120 minutes). Six were completed within 30 minutes, 13 within 1 hour, 5 within 75 minutes, and 1 in 2 hours.

This early experience taught me that (1) laparoscopic cholecystectomy is feasible, (2) the operating time is acceptable although initially longer than that with open cholecystectomy, (3) many patients can be treated on an ambulatory basis, and (4) pain and discomfort are less and convalescence is shorter than with open cholecystectomy.

Since then, I have performed laparoscopic cholecystectomy in 275 other patients. There have been no deaths and few complications have occurred. The complications encountered have been with the "difficult" cholecystectomies, and my experience with these cases is responsible for modifications in technique.

An unrecognized problem was a cholecystoduodenal fistula in a patient in whom the duodenum was adherent to the midbody of the gallbladder. This adhesion was dissected by removing a rim of gallbladder wall. No fistula was evident. An EndoLoop was placed on the duodenal wall. The patient was informed in the recovery room that the cystic duct appeared dilated intraoperatively and a small cholecystoduodenal fistula and common duct stones could be present. She was observed for several hours postoperatively. She experienced unanticipated pain and tachycardia. The operative site was explored through a Band-Aid incision; a 2 mm cholecystoduodenal fistula was found and the distal common duct was noted to be impacted with calculi. The stones were removed from the common duct, the fistula was extended, and a choledochoduodenostomy was performed. The patient was dismissed on the fourth postoperative day. The possibility that the biliary tree was chronically decompressed through the fistula was suspected.

Three patients with gangrenous cholecystitis or severely inflamed gallbladders developed subhepatic collections, which were drained percutaneously.

Two required readmission for 2 and 6 days, respectively. Since then we have emphasized the need for thorough irrigation of the subhepatic space at surgery and administration of systemic antibiotics for several days. This practice has greatly reduced the incidence of this complication.

Two patients required hepaticojejunostomy. In one, a stone impacted in the infundibulum caused erosion of the wall of the hepatic duct. This condition was seen at laparoscopy and a roux limb was used to close the defect. The second patient had an anomalous entrance of the upper duct system into the gallbladder: the exiting duct from the gallbladder emptied directly into the duodenum. This rarest of biliary anomalies was recognized only postoperatively by the observation of persistent bile drainage. A roux limb was used to reconnect the small upper ducts, but a stricture developed within 3 months that required further treatment. Both cases prompted me to institute the practice of ascertaining the integrity of the upper duct system by visual inspection at laparoscopy supplemented by cholangiography when necessary. Moving the camera to the fundic port provides improved visualization in this situation. These patients were treated early in my experience with difficult cholecystectomies.

One patient had abdominal tenderness postoperatively; a biliary isotope scan showed bile leakage with no flow of isotope into the duodenum. At laparoscopic surgery the cystic duct–common duct junction was clearly identified and a clip seemed to have completely occluded the cystic duct. Exploration through a Band-Aid incision revealed a bile leak through an accessory duct at the dome of the liver, which was cauterized.

Two patients had bleeding. One patient with a known coagulopathy had a qualitative platelet defect. The laparoscopic cholecystectomy was converted to an open procedure and the patient required blood and coagulation factors over the next 48 hours.

One other patient had a difficult dissection that required lysing of adhesions and open control of a bleeding vessel in the liver bed. Three other patients required conversion to open procedures. In one the gallbladder was obscured by the stomach and was never seen laparoscopically. An imminent cholecystogastric fistula was suspected. A second patient had multiple operations and despite adequate pneumoperitoneum and camera insertion being achieved, the 5 mm operating ports could not be seen. The patient underwent a Band-Aid cholecystectomy and was dismissed 24 hours later. The third patient had a deeply embedded gallbladder, and the clamps were ineffective in holding the gallbladder wall. This case antedated the arrival of a full instrument set, so open cholecystectomy was performed. One patient with known duodenal ulcer disease developed a spontaneous perforating ulcer 48 hours postoperatively. This defect was plicated and was technically unrelated to the cholecystectomy.

Thus overall morbidity was 4%; 2.6% required laparotomy. In the last 200 cases, there have been no duct injuries or bile leaks and only two patients (adhesions, gastric fistula) required conversion to an open procedure. Difficult gallbladders currently constitute 30% to 40% of my referral practice. With increased experience, the operating team functions more efficiently. Currently operations for chronic cholecystitis are routinely done in less than 20 minutes (without cholangiography). Difficult gallbladders require 30 to 60 minutes.

REFERENCES

1. Conn H. Therapeutic portocaval anastomoses: To shunt or not to shunt. Gastroenterology 67:1065-1071, 1974.
2. Cuschieri A, Dubois F, Mouiel J, et al. The European experience with laparoscopic cholecystectomy. Am J Surg 161(3):385-387, 1991.
3. Berci G, Sacker JM. The Los Angeles experience with laparoscopic cholecystectomy. Am J Surg 161(3):382-384, 1991.
4. Voyles CR, Petro AB, Meena AL, et al. A practical approach to laparoscopic cholecystectomy. Am J Surg 161(3):365-370, 1991.
5. The Southern Surgeons Club. A prospective analysis of 1518 cholecystectomies. N Engl J Med 324:1073-1078, 1991.
6. Airan MA. Report on presentation at the Society of American Gastrointestinal Endoscopic Surgeons. Gen Surg News, July 1991; personal communication, August 1991.
7. Flowers JL, Bailey RW, Scovill WA, et al. The Baltimore experience with laparoscopic management of acute cholecystitis. Am J Surg 161(3):388-392, 1991.
8. Reddick EJ, Olsen D, Spaw A, et al. Safe performance of difficult laparoscopic cholecystectomies. Am J Surg 161(3):377-381, 1991.
9. Vitale GC, Collet D, Larson GM, et al. Interruption of professional and home activity after laparoscopic cholecystectomy among French and American patients. Am J Surg 161(3):396-398, 1991.

10. Spaw AT, Reddick EJ, Olsen DO. Outpatient laparoscopic laser cholecystectomy: Analysis of 500 procedures. Surg Laparos Endosc 1:2-7, 1991.

11. Cooperman AM. Laparoscopic cholecystectomy—Report on 90 cases. Am J Gastroenterol (in press).

12. Philips EH, Berci G, Carroll B, et al. The importance of intraoperative cholangiography during laparoscopic cholecystectomy. Am Surg 56:792-795, 1990.

13. Graves H Jr, Ballinger JF, Anderson WJ. Appraisal of laparoscopic cholecystectomy. Ann Surg 213:655-664, 1991.

14. Soper NJ. Laparoscopic cholecystectomy. Curr Probl Surg 28(9):644, 1991.

15. Rubio PA, Rowe G, Feste JR. Endoscopic laser cholecystectomy: Initial report. J Clin Laser Med Surg 23-26, 1990.

16. Zucker KA, Bailey RW, Gadacz TR, et al. Laparoscopic guided cholecystectomy: A plea for cautious enthusiasm. Am J Surg 161:36-44, 1991.

17. Peters JH, Ellison EC, Innes JT, et al. Safety and efficacy of laparoscopic cholecystectomy. A prospective analysis of 100 initial patients. Ann Surg 213(1):3-12, 1991.

Index